OFFICE PRACTICE OF SKIN SURGERY

BRYAN C. SCHULTZ, M.D.

Assistant Clinical Professor of Medicine
(Dermatology), Loyola University, Maywood, Illinois

PETER McKINNEY, M.D.

Professor of Plastic Surgery,
Northwestern University, Chicago, Illinois

1985

W. B. SAUNDERS COMPANY

Philadelphia / London / Toronto / Mexico City / Rio de Janeiro / Sydney / Tokyo

W. B. Saunders Company: West Washington Square
Philadelphia, PA 19105

1 St. Anne's Road
Eastbourne, East Sussex BN21 3UN, England

1 Goldthorne Avenue
Toronto, Ontario M8Z 5T9, Canada

Apartado 26370—Cedro 512
Mexico 4, D.F., Mexico

Rua Coronel Cabrita, 8
Sao Cristovao Caixa Postal 21176
Rio de Janeiro, Brazil

9 Waltham Street
Artarmon, N.S.W. 2064, Australia

Ichibancho, Central Bldg., 22-1 Ichibancho
Chiyoda-Ku, Tokyo 102, Japan

Library of Congress Cataloging in Publication Data

Schultz, Bryan C.

Office practice of skin surgery.

1. Skin—Surgery.   2. Surgery, Outpatient. I. McKinney,
Peter.   II. Title. [DNLM: 1. Ambulatory Surgery.   2.
Skin—surgery. WR 650 S387o]

RD520.S38 1985   617'.477   84–14022

ISBN 0–7216–1326–8

Office Practice of Skin Surgery   ISBN   0–7216–1326–8

Last digit is the print number: 9   8   7   6   5   4   3   2   1

*To my wife Cathy and my children Carrie, Megan, and Erin,
for their love and inspiration.*

Dr. Schultz

To my colleagues.

Dr. McKinney

Preface

This book is written for the practicing dermatologist, housestaff, general practitioners, and other physicians who perform many common surgical procedures on the skin. It should prove helpful in quickly obtaining practical information concerning aesthetic results in common surgical procedures of the skin.

This text takes a different approach than do plastic surgery books and most skin surgery texts written for dermatologists, in that we present a regional and a pathological approach. One section deals specifically with the surgical treatment of skin lesions in different regions (e.g., eye, nose, hand). Generally, defects that can be closed by simple advancement techniques are the topic of discussion in this regional approach rather than major reconstructive challenges, which are better left for the plastic surgeon. Another section discusses the most common skin lesions by pathological diagnosis with an emphasis on aesthetic results (e.g., nevi, epidermal cysts, seborrheic keratoses, basal cell carcinoma).

This regional and pathological approach will give the practitioner an easy reference for specific skin lesions in specific areas. For example, in considering a 0.4 cm nevus on the nose, a reference to nevi in the pathological section and the nose in the regional section will provide practical information needed.

Advances in techniques, suture materials, dressings, and assorted instruments allow for better aesthetic results for even the simplest surgical skin procedures. An introductory section discusses the outpatient facility, instruments, preoperative evaluation, anesthesia, suturing, and wound dressings. An appendix shows photos of some common equipment and instruments helpful in doing office surgery.

We hope that the co-authorship of a plastic surgeon and a dermatologist will provide a broader viewpoint of skin surgery. The plastic surgeon offers the focus to enable the reader to achieve maximum aesthetic surgical results. The dermatologist handles the many practical problems of the large number of skin lesions presented to him daily in an office setting.

Techniques most likely to give superior cosmetic results are stressed, but alternative modalities are mentioned. The authors by training and experience have a clear preference for excisional surgery in many circumstances, but fully recognize that other techniques may be quite acceptable when performed by physicians frequently using them.

BRYAN C. SCHULTZ
PETER MCKINNEY

Contents

PART 4 A Pathologic Approach to Surgery of Common Skin Lesions

PART 1

Introduction
to
Skin Surgery

chapter 1

THE OUTPATIENT SKIN SURGERY SUITE AND SURGICAL INSTRUMENTS

Most offices can easily have one room set up for excisional skin surgery. It is preferable to have this room used exclusively for surgery of the skin. If this is not possible, meticulous attention to cleaning of all surfaces within the room is mandatory. Personnel circulating in this room should be clothed in proper surgical attire and should not be wearing laboratory jackets or other clothing that could be contaminated from other patients.

Patients known to be carrying pathogenic bacteria or viruses (for example, patients with herpes simplex, abscesses, or impetigo) should be kept out of the room. This is especially true if the operating room is located in a busy general or dermatologic practice. Patients with generalized skin disease such as atopic eczema and psoriasis are known to frequently harbor coagulase-positive staphylococci. Patients with these diseases or with draining, crusting lesions should be kept out of the room. Common sense dictates that drainage of furuncles, acne cysts, infected epidermal cysts, and so on should not be done in this room.

It is best that the room to be used for surgery be located in an area of low traffic flow. The room should have a separate entrance and exit and should not serve as a thoroughfare to another room. There should be adequate space, ventilation, and cooling at all times in the surgery room. This becomes extremely important for both patient and physician, since active perspiration by the patient during the procedure from excessive heat may lead to extreme discomfort and possible contamination of the wound. Adequate ventilation and proper positioning are necessary for patients with cardiorespiratory problems. It should be remembered that if the physician uses only one assistant, three people (i.e., physician, assistant, and patient) will be confined to a small area for a prolonged period.

A cool light source should always be used, since lighting contributes to increased temperature in the operative area. High quality surgical lighting, preferably mounted on the ceiling and having a sterilizable handle, should be used. There are acceptable floor stand models, but these can become cumbersome in certain situations and may interfere with the mobility of the physician or his assistant. Spotlight-type surgical lamps may shed brilliant light that can interfere with the surgeon's perception by blinding his vision or by casting deep shadows in portions of the surgical field. It is advisable to talk to a physician who has used a similar light prior to purchasing any expensive surgical lighting device.

The single most important piece of equipment is the operating table. A power table with adjustable articulating headrest and footrest is preferable. Separate controls for table height, head elevation, and preferably foot elevation should be included. Such controls may be built into the head of the table itself or may be available as a foot control. A foot control is preferable because it enables the surgeon to adjust the table himself during surgery. Ideally, the table should be capable of being rapidly placed in a Trendelenburg position. The surface of the table should be easily washable and preferably should accommodate a paper roll. Some dental and podiatry chairs will not accommodate a paper roll; these chairs may also have stitching that could become stained with blood. Small potential problems such as these should be considered and checked before a power table is purchased.

Some tables are equipped to rotate 180 degrees on their base, but this feature is not needed in most offices. The physician may find that operating from a sitting position is most comfortable or most appropriate in certain circumstances. The table should therefore be adjustable to the appropriate height. The surgeon may also prefer a table with a head piece narrower than the rest of the table to permit easy accessibility to the head and neck area, especially if he does cosmetic procedures frequently.

If purchase of a chair-type table is being considered, several factors should be scrutinized. A table may be well suited for surgery in the area of the face but have a permanent curvature in the area of the trunk, causing that area to be flexed during surgery. Such a curvature would also make the prone position uncomfortable or impossible. Some tables also have a permanently attached foot rest that is perpendicular to the table, making surgery of the foot on these tables almost impossible.

One dental chair that is particularly good for office surgery is the Pelton Crane Coachman. This chair is extremely comfortable for patients and will recline completely, allowing for surgery with the patient in a horizontal position without significant curvature of the torso. It may even be placed in a slight Trendelenburg position. This feature also allows the patient to lie comfortably on his stomach, a problem when a fixed-contour curvature is present in a power chair. Armrests swing out readily for access to any area. A good articulating headrest is an available option. A unique power switch enables the operator to raise or lower the chair base and back at the same time with one finger. Foot control is also available. With one touch of a button the chair will descend and return to the sitting position automatically. A more expensive model can be programmed to assume automatically any position the operator desires. Chair-mounting posts may hold any dental light, but such lighting is a small, restricted horizontal band that will not illuminate evenly a whole face at once and therefore may be inappropriate for some skin surgery.

A disadvantage of the Pelton Crane dental chair is the need to add extra upholstery or other insulation to the bottom of the arms. The exposed metal on the undersurface could transmit electrosurgical current through the patient's hand, especially if a good grounding plate is not used. This alteration is a simple procedure, however, for a chair that patients describe as extremely comfortable.

Another popular chair-type table is the Dexta table. Although it is considerably more expensive, it is an excellent table. It is available in a narrower model that permits easy access to the center of the torso during surgery. If the surgeon operates with his back bent even two inches more than normal for any period of time, back fatigue will be considerably increased. This factor is not a minor point, and it is unfortunate that many office procedure/surgery tables are considerably wider than standard operating tables. It is important to compare table width before buying. The Dexta table has optional stirrups, intravenous pole, and arm boards that are not available with the Pelton Crane dental chair.

It is preferable to have a tile floor in the surgical area for easy cleaning. Shelving and other surfaces should be washable for cleaning and disinfection. Stainless steel tables and shelving are preferable but not necessary. A Mayo stand of adjustable height should be placed close to the operating area. Medications for intravenous, intramuscular, and local infiltration may be located on shelving close to the operating area. Any chemical cauterants or hemostatic agents should be placed far enough away that they cannot spill into the operative area. A full bottle of sterile eye wash should be close at hand in case an irritating substance gets into the patient's eye.

The surgical sink should have a faucet placed well above the sink itself, allowing the physician to scrub and rinse freely under running water. Disposable, sterile surgical scrub brushes with appropriate impregnated disinfectant should be available above the sink area. Either foot pedals or a knee control is preferable for the surgical sink. Sterile towels may be handed to the physician at the time of surgery. These may be contained in the surgical pack or packaged separately.

THE SURGICAL PACK

The following are some general suggestions for a standard surgical pack to be used during routine surgery of the skin. Many additions (especially instruments) may be made to such a pack. Instrument type and size depend largely on the personal preference of the operator.

The surgical pack may be wrapped in suitable cloth material (for example surgical towels) or in autoclave paper and closed with autoclave tape. The autoclave tape will turn the appropriate color when sterilization is complete, as an added check on sterilization. Optional colored autoclave tape may be used for coding packs, and the tape may also be written on to describe the contents.

The surgical pack may be sterilized with steam under pressure in the autoclave. A separate sharp instrument pack may be sterilized with dry heat to avoid dulling sharp edges. The latter technique requires the use of a metal instrument tray or wrapping the instruments in metal foil (e.g., aluminum foil). A sterile transfer forceps is then used to transfer instruments to the open sterile autoclaved pack. (We autoclave all instruments in the surgical pack for convenience.)

The following is a list of recommended materials to be contained in the surgical pack (Fig. 1–1) to be autoclaved under steam pressure:

1. An adequate number of 2 × 2 or 4 × 4 sponges
2. A pointed wooden tooth pick for drawing the line of excision
3. A glass 5-cc syringe (optional). A disposable syringe may be added at the time of surgery.
4. Towel drapes (if sterile disposable fenestrated drapes are not used)
5. Four or more towel clamps (if towel drapes are used)
6. A No. 3 Bard-Parker scalpel handle with centimeter markings on one side
7. A 4½ inch (Webster or Ryder type) smooth jaw needle holder. Note that the jaw of the Ryder is narrower, allowing more needle exposure when passing small precision point needles through tissue.
8. Two or three short, curved mosquito hemostats
9. A small glass or metal medicine cup for marking dye (optional)
10. A small tissue forceps with medium 1 × 2 teeth (e.g., Adson or Castro-Viello type)
11. One forceps without teeth
12. One or two skin hooks (optional)
13. One dissecting scissors (optional)

The following are sharp instruments that may be sterilized by dry heat to prevent dulling, if preferred:

1. One short, curved, sharp iris scissors
2. One straight suture scissors

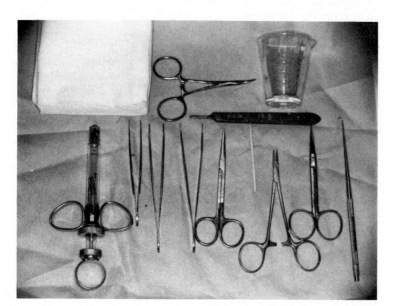

FIGURE 1–1. Surgical pack.

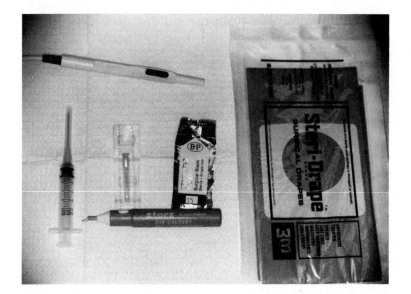

FIGURE 1–2. Sterile items that may be added to the surgical pack.

The following may be added to the open surgical pack at the time of surgery (Fig. 1–2):

1.   Disposable plastic 5-cc syringes with attached 18-gauge needle
2.   A 30-gauge needle (this may be attached after anesthetic is drawn up in the 18-gauge needle)
3.   Disposable fenestrated drape with adhesive backing (e.g., 3-M Steridrape), clear or blue
4.   A No. 15 Bard-Parker blade
5.   A disposable hot cautery unit (e.g., Concept Unit) (optional)
6.   Handle for electrocoagulator (if used for electrocoagulation of blood vessels, a ground plate should always be placed under the patient)
7.   Appropriate absorbable and nonabsorbable sutures
8.   Sterile methylene blue or gentian violet may be added to the medicine cup at the time of surgery.

THE EMERGENCY KIT

One of the most important items for any medical office, whether office surgery is done there or not, is an adequate emergency kit. All physicians should have had extensive training in CPR and should routinely refresh their memories by mock sessions if they do not perform CPR regularly. In a day when even nonmedical personnel are trained extensively in CPR, the staff of physician's office should serve as an example of a well-trained unit. A myocardial infarction or cardiac arrhythmia may occur in the physician's office, totally unrelated to any therapy or surgery being done. The physician's staff should be thoroughly trained in dealing with such an emergency.

The primary goal during any emergency is to maintain vital functions until the patient can be transported to a proper hospital facility. If surgery is done in the office, phone numbers for the best paramedical ambulance teams in the area should be available at all phones. Staff members should have well-defined duties in case of emergency. We will not attempt to cover the broad field of emergency medicine but simply make some recommendations as to the essentials of an emergency kit. The following items may be contained in an emergency kit for the office:

EMERGENCY KIT

1. Oxygen supply system
2. "Ambu" bag with adult and pediatric masks and tubing for connection to oxygen system
3. Intravenous equipment
   A. Tourniquet
   B. Angiocath or Intracath tubing with 18-gauge needles
   C. Tape and arm board
   D. IV tubing and 500-ml bags of normal saline and D5W
   E. Small excision kit for possible "cut-down" to obtain an adequate vein
4. Medications
   A. Sodium bicarbonate—prepackaged 50-ml syringes (at least two)
   B. Epinephrine 1:1000 (1-ml ampule) for allergic reactions
                         1:10,000 (10-ml ampule with intracardiac needle)
   C. 50% dextrose (50-ml ampules) for hypoglycemic reactions
   D. Lidocaine 2 per cent (5-ml syringe—100 mg)
   E. Aminophylline (10-ml (250 mg) ampules)
   F. Narcan (10 ml (0.4 mg/ml))—only if narcotics are used before or during surgery
   G. Valium (10-mg ampule for IV use)—for epilepsy
   H. Benadryl (50-mg ampule)

When only plain lidocaine is being used as an anesthetic during skin surgery, cardiorespiratory complications directly due to surgery are highly unlikely. Blood loss should be minimal. History should rule out the extremely rare true allergic reaction to lidocaine. In these circumstances there is no more risk of cardiorespiratory emergency than that encountered in a dentist's office. In fact, since skin surgery should be painless, the psychologic stress factor should be less than in a dentist's office or a court of law.

Careful analysis of relative risk, therefore, does not dictate a need for EKG equipment or defibrillators. To put this in perspective, it is not practical to have such equipment everywhere a person possibly under some emotional stress (such as skin surgery) is in close proximity to a person capable of using a defibrillator. Extensive procedures with the use of multiple drugs for anesthesia may be more easily and appropriately done in a facility that routinely handles such cases.

chapter 2

PREOPERATIVE EVALUATION AND PREPARATION OF THE PATIENT

A good history and physical examination are essential to the preoperative evaluation of any surgical patient. For office or outpatient surgery, an extensive questionnaire is often helpful in evaluating the patient. This questionnaire may contain any current symptomatology; a detailed past history of procedures performed, with dates and reasons for the procedures; past hospitalizations; a good family history with specific questions concerning bleeding disorders and cardiovascular disorders; all current medications; any history of allergies (especially to local anesthetic); and the date of the most recent complete physical examination.

The patient may also be questioned specifically concerning any history of epilepsy, since it is possible to precipitate convulsions with larger doses of anesthetic. If electrocoagulation is to be used during surgery, the patient should be questioned about a cardiac pacemaker. This is particularly a problem with demand-type pacemakers, since the electrical current may falsely indicate the presence of a heart beat to the electronic pacemaker. In this situation the pacemaker will not electrically induce a cardiac contraction that may be needed.

Although frequently ignored, a complete examination of the entire skin surface prior to surgery may uncover other bacterial, viral, or fungal disease in areas distant from the surgical site. The physician may elect to simply question the patient concerning symptoms of such infections. Although infections need not be absolute contraindications to skin surgery at a different location, adequate precautions must be taken. Likewise the patient may be questioned as to symptomatology indicating infection of the upper respiratory, gastrointestinal, and genitourinary systems. If surgery is to be done in the facial or genital area, the patient

9

may be questioned about a history of herpes simplex in these areas. The physician and patient should be aware of the fact that the trauma of surgery in an area where recurrent herpes simplex has been a problem may precipitate the herpetic infection in that area. The development of a herpetic infection in the area of surgery can result in a poor cosmetic result. This is especially true in the perioral region. The patient should also be told to report any herpetic infection developing between the time of the preoperative visit and surgery. In fact, specific instructions should be given to the patient to report *any* infection or other physical ailment developing between the time of the preoperative visit and the scheduled surgery.

Blood pressure, pulse, and respiratory rate may be taken at the preoperative visit and also immediately prior to surgery. This is more important when using epinephrine in the anesthetic. Plain lidocaine in small amounts locally infiltrated should not affect these parameters. Blood pressure is especially important, since hypertensive patients may bleed profusely, especially when undergoing surgery of the scalp or other vascular areas. Special note should be made of any irregularities in pulse, especially in older patients. These patients may have multiple PVC's or atrial fibrillation unknown to them or their family physician, whom they may not have seen for several years.

Any medications, either prescription or nonprescription, should be brought to the attention of the physician. Anticoagulants and especially any aspirin-containing remedies may make surgery more difficult by causing profuse bleeding. This is especially of interest if epinephrine is not used with local anesthetic infiltration. Many small procedures may frequently be performed even with prolonged bleeding times, but this requires careful evaluation of the risk of hematoma or bleeding and their consequences in the area to be operated on.

The patient should be warned to avoid any aspirin or aspirin-containing products for at least seven to ten days prior to the procedure. The patient and physician should be aware of the fact that as little as one aspirin tablet will induce the maximum bleeding defect. Depending upon the severity of pain the patient may use acetaminophen or acetaminophen with codeine. If skin surgery is anticipated to be quite vascular, as with extensive scalp surgery, avoiding aspirin-containing products may be quite important; however, if the procedure is limited and aspirin-containing products for the management of arthritis or other severe inflammatory disorders are necessary, these products may be continued in most circumstances.

Cardiac medications, antihypertensive medications, and antiarrhythmic medications should be carefully reviewed. The patient should be specifically instructed to continue these medications. This may be in contrast to what is done for procedures under general anesthesia.

Except for some concern for occasional problem bleeding, most skin surgery can be performed while the patient continues to take all of his current medications. Diabetics who are on hypoglycemic agents or insulin should be questioned concerning appropriate meal time. If this falls during probable surgery time, it may be better to reschedule the surgical time rather than change routine medication times.

Blood testing should probably be done prior to *some* minor surgical procedures. If recent testing has been done by the patient's general physician, it may be helpful to obtain results from him. A CBC with differential, a fasting chemistry screen, and a coagulation profile may be in order. A prothrombin time (PT), partial thromboplastin time (PTT), bleeding time, and platelet count should be sufficient for most patients without a family history of coagulation disorders. These are usually needed only with extensive or particularly vascular skin surgery.

With more vascular procedures and especially procedures that may spray blood (for example, hair transplantation with power punch and dermabrasion), the physician may want to order a test of hepatitis surface antigen. Questions as to previous hepatitis and possible recent contact, along with screening of liver enzymes on the chemistry screen, should identify many patients recently infected as well as possible chronic carriers. Physicians doing frequent skin surgery should consider immunization of themselves with the new hepatitis B vaccine. This is especially true for those using frequent electrosurgery where blood droplets spatter far enough to reach mucosal surfaces of the eye, nose, and mouth. This is a good reason to use a mask even for minor electrosurgery.

For most routine surgery of the skin the patient does not have to scrub with an antibacterial agent prior to surgery. The surgical area should be thoroughly washed the night before the procedure. Allow the patient to have a light breakfast with juice on the morning of the procedure. This can prevent hypoglycemia. Unlike general anesthesia, vomiting is not a problem with local infiltration anesthesia. The patient should avoid any caffeinated beverages on the day of the procedure, since they may precipitate hypertension or arrhythmias.

SKIN DISINFECTION AND PROTECTION OF SURGICAL PERSONNEL

Disinfection of surgical personnel and the surgical site before skin surgery must take into account both resident and transient bacterial flora, regional variation in bacterial populations and density, available scrubs and disinfecting agents, and sterile protective coverings. There is no doubt that with most general surgery more meticulous attention to scrub technique, disinfection of the skin, and sterile protective surgical wear have led to a dramatic decrease in postoperative wound infections; however, when performing limited procedures on the skin, many physicians question the necessity for sterile technique as rigid as that used in a standard operating room. Perhaps one way of assessing the effectiveness of aseptic surgical technique is to record any postoperative wound infection and to compute an approximate percentage infection rate. This rate should usually not be greater than 0.1 per cent (1 per 1000).

In our office surgical rooms, an estimated 3000 minor surgical procedures are performed each year. Approximately 1500 to 2000 procedures require sutures. Infection rate (small amount of pus, fever, or localized erythema and induration) is *at most* 0.03 to 0.08 per cent (one or two infections per year). Serious infections (cellulitis, copious pus, lymphangitis, etc.) are almost never seen. For approximately the last 7500 surgical procedures we have used plain 70 per cent isopropyl alcohol cleansing of the surgical site, except for using povidone-iodine (Betadine) in the genital area, perirectal area, lower legs, and feet. Application of dry sterile postoperative dressings (e.g., gauze) and gentle

TABLE 2–1. POST-SUTURE SURGERY INSTRUCTIONS FOR PATIENTS

Steri-Strips have been placed on the surgical site. They should remain in place until the next appointment. *If* they do come off, follow *all* instructions below.
OR
Steri-Strips have *not* been placed on the surgical site, so follow *all* directions below.
1. Cleanse area *gently* with 70% isopropyl alcohol one or two times a day and cover with a sterile Telfa pad or gauze (just enough to cover the wound). Keep in place with nonallergenic Dermicel or paper tape. Do not use plain adhesive bandage strips after the first day; they get too sticky.
2. If soreness or pain is a problem, use cold compresses or acetaminophen tablets every four to six hours.
3. If there is redness or significant swelling more than ½ inch beyond the suture line or pus draining from the wound, call the doctor. A small amount of superficial crust or scab, however, is normal. Take your temperature two times daily (A.M. and P.M.). If it is greater than 100°F (it will always be somewhat higher in late afternoon and evening) call the doctor, since this *may* indicate wound infection.
4. The area should not be immersed in water for the first five to seven days. When bathing, attempt to avoid the surgery area during that time.

cleansing with H_2O_2 or alcohol have been standard postoperative written directions (Table 2–1). One mild infection resulted from a wide excision of basal cell carcinoma on the forehead. Extensive undermining and electrocautery for hemostasis was necessary. Erythromycin 1 gm per day cleared the infection rapidly. I recently tried a new clear adhesive dressing in a patient with multiple excised dysplastic nevi. Multiple areas of draining pus developed in surgical sites on the trunk. This responded well to erythromycin. Since our last wound infection had been almost two years before this (the patient with basal cell carcinoma of the forehead mentioned above), we will probably not use occlusive "breathing" dressings again unless infection rates change for some unforeseen reason. This is anecdotal information, of course, but it may be of interest or value to some readers.

The surgical scrub is important in removing transient bacterial flora, which account for most pathogenic bacteria present on the skin. The surgeon should scrub for five to ten minutes before the first surgery of the day. The use of a brush and a fingernail cleaner are helpful. Fingernails should be kept short, so that only a maximum of 1 mm of nail is projecting distally. If the surgeon has a tendency to develop severe irritation or allergic reaction from scrubbing, it is advisable to scrub only to the wrist rather than to the elbow. If the skin becomes chronically excoriated and a subsequent dermatitis ensues, the skin is more likely to carry pathogens.

Agents available for use as surgical scrubs are iodophors, hexachlorophene compounds, chlorhexidine compounds, and regular soaps. Iodophors are the most commonly used agents, with chlorhexidine compounds gaining more acceptance in recent years. Either standard latex surgical gloves or various brands of hypoallergenic gloves (some made of vinyl) should be used. Hands affected with a mild dermatitis may populate with pathogens and cause a much increased infection rate. Chlorhexidine (Hibiclens) is less irritating to the skin than most iodophors.

Most suture skin surgery should be performed with a face mask. If the hair is short and clean a hair covering is not mandatory, but it is preferred. If there is a recent documented postoperative wound infection with *Staphylococcus aureus*, it is a good habit to take nasal cultures of personnel assisting with skin surgery. It may be found that one of the staff members is a carrier of S. aureus. In most situations of minor surgery of the skin a complete gowning technique is not necessary. It is quite obvious, however, that contaminated clothing should be kept out of the surgery room. The use of scrub suits is encouraged so that clean, noncontaminated clothes are present in the surgical room.

When cleansing the operative site, perhaps the most important factor is the mechanical cleaning, removing most of the transient bacterial flora. As mentioned before, transient flora are more likely to carry pathogens than are resident flora. One prospective study by two plastic surgeons showed that preparation of the skin with physiologic saline solution only resulted in an infection rate of less than 1 per cent in 807 consecutive cases. The authors suggested that gentle cleansing was adequate, provided that meticulous attention was given to the handling of tissues during surgery. Iodophors, 70 per cent isopropyl alcohol, and chlorhexidine all seem to be acceptable cleansing agents for skin preparation before minor skin surgery. Areas where skin surfaces provide an occlusive atmosphere should be cleansed for a longer period of time. In areas such as the toe webs, the groin, and the lower leg and in patients with vascular compromise, a long-acting iodophor preparation may be preferable.

During surgery the operative site should be protected with either sterile towels and towel clamps or disposable fenestrated sterile fields. One such field is the Steridrape by 3-M (see Fig. 1–2). This drape may be obtained with an adhesive backing so that only the surgical area is exposed during surgery. It is available in blue or clear. Blood or other liquid draining from the operative site will drain down the Steridrape (if adhesive backing is used) rather than under a sterile towel and onto the patient. This improves patient comfort and makes surgery much easier near orifices. It also makes cleaning up after surgery much easier. It is helpful to have a sterile handle for a ceiling surgical light so that the surgeon may move the light during the procedure. This may not be necessary if there is a circulating assistant present.

chapter 3

ANESTHESIA

Anesthesia for office skin surgery is administered almost entirely by local injection. The use of inhalation anesthesia entails risks that may not be easily controlled in a small outpatient surgical room.

One distinct advantage of local anesthesia of the skin is that it is almost always possible to perform a completely painless surgical procedure.

NEEDLES

For initial skin penetration we prefer never to use anything larger than a 30-gauge needle. There is no question that 25- and even 27-gauge needles draw a significantly greater painful response from patients. With children, one may sometimes demonstrate how the tiny needle can penetrate the skin and feel similar to a "mosquito" rather than a real needle. After initial penetration and injection of a small amount of anesthetic, larger needles may be introduced if necessary for slow infiltration distal to the initial site. Rarely is this use of larger needles necessary for small procedures.

If the needles are also to be used for electrocoagulation at other times (e.g., telangiectatic blood vessels), there are two options: (1) A metal-based needle directly mounted on an appropriate electrocoagulating handle may be used. (2) A plastic-based needle (e.g., B-D type) may be held by the operator's bare hand (the plastic will not conduct current). Any standard electrocoagulating needle touched to the metal shaft of this needle will then direct current to the patient.

Thirty-gauge needles may also be obtained for the dental type syringes (e.g., Cook-Waite type) with 1.8-cc Carpules. These may not, however, be used with electrocoagulating devices.

SYRINGES

Plastic disposable, glass, and stainless steel dental-type syringes may be used. The operator exerts less pressure when using a syringe with a smaller diameter. Plastic syringes larger than 3 cc are difficult to use with 30-gauge needles for this reason. Even with 3-cc syringes, it is advisable to get syringes with adequate flanges (e.g., B-D Luer-Lok tip)

15

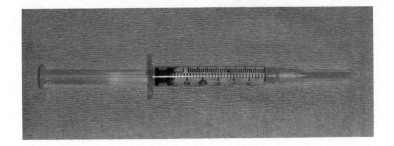

FIGURE 3–1. This plastic 3-cc syringe has adequate flanges for easy counterpressure during injection.

for exerting counterpressure with the index and middle fingers while injecting with the thumb (Fig. 3–1).

Glass syringes usually come with a circular attachment to the plunger that facilitates the application of pressure while preventing the thumb from slipping (Fig. 3–2). The disadvantage of these is their short life expectancy with repeated autoclaving. After extensive use the plunger may not slide as smoothly, and eventually it begins to stick.

Dental-type syringes that receive 1.8-cc anesthetic Carpules are perhaps the easiest to use. The extremely small diameter of the Carpule makes injection very easy. These syringes should be obtained with the optional hook that punctures the rubber plunger of the Carpule (e.g., Cook-Waite aspirator syringe), allowing for aspiration during injection (Fig. 3–3). A disadvantage to the use of Carpules is a more limited selection of anesthetic concentration (e.g., usually not available in 0.5 per cent or 1 per cent plain lidocaine). Also, re-autoclaving is time consuming. Plastic syringes are disposable.

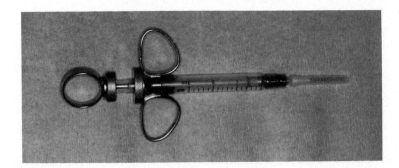

FIGURE 3–2. This glass syringe with a ring for thumb pressure is easy to use. Re-autoclaving is necessary and results in a relatively short useful lifespan.

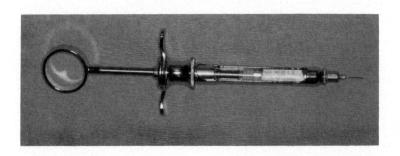

FIGURE 3–3. This dental-type syringe has a spear-shaped plunger that penetrates the rubber plunger in disposable Carpules. This construction enables the operator to aspirate with this type of syringe.

JET INJECTORS

Several special circumstances make the jet injectors useful instruments. Anesthetic is injected into the skin by a high-velocity, thin, streamed jet, usually propelled by a powerful spring within the device. The depth of injection is about 4 mm but may vary significantly depending upon tissue consistency and the jet device itself. Careful consideration of underlying structures is necessary before using the jet device. Use of a jet device on one patient for injecting corticosteroid into lichen planus of the buccal mucosa resulted in complete penetration through the cheek (at least 1 cm thickness). This could theoretically result in intraneural injection (e.g., facial nerve) and possible neuritis.

For anesthetizing areas in children, the slower needle injection and infiltration method may not be acceptable. This is especially true of the child who cannot be kept immobile. The needle may come out repeatedly before the injection is complete. Multiple quick jets can be used in rapid succession, even if the child is uncooperative. It is helpful (but optional) here to use epinephrine with the anesthetic for prolonged action. The child may then be transferred to another area for the surgical procedure. This allows time and a change in surroundings to quiet the child. The procedure can then be painless and easier to perform. Also, more anesthetic may be infiltrated (if needed) through the anesthetized wheals created with the jet injector.

For areas where injection may be painful during the entire infiltration time, a jet injector has the advantage of rapid, split-second injection. The periungual area is such a location, and jet injection is extremely useful here. Two injections are usually all that is needed for anesthesia of the proximal periungual area (Fig. 3–4).

When multiple small areas must be anesthetized (e.g., multiple

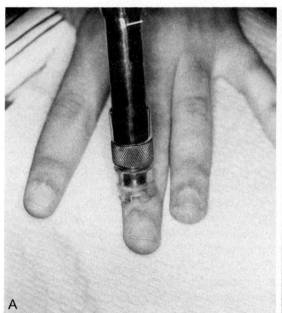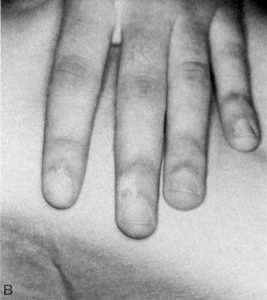

A   B

FIGURE 3–4. *A*, Positioning the Dermojet to anesthetize the periungual area with 1 per cent lidocaine. *B*, Wheal created by jet injection.

small warts), the jet injector may be preferred by patients. If one area larger than a few millimeters is to be anesthetized, however, multiple jet injections are needed. With larger single areas one needle injection followed by slow advancing infiltration is usually preferable.

Jet injectors are also useful in the patient who is clearly terrified by needles, but will accept the quick sting of the jet injector. If a larger area is to be anesthetized in such a patient, a dermal wheal is raised with the jet injector first. Subsequent slow infiltration with the long needle advancing from the wheal will prevent the patient from experiencing the sensation of being stuck with a needle.

ANESTHETIC

The most commonly used local anesthetics are classified in the amide and ester groups. Amide anesthetics (e.g., lidocaine, carbocaine) have a much lower incidence of true allergic reaction than those in the ester group (e.g., procaine). Also, patients who have been sensitized topically to para-amino benzoic products (e.g., benzocaine products, PABA sunscreens) may cross-sensitize to the ester group of anesthetics.

True allergy to lidocaine is probably rare. In some instances it may be related to the preservative rather than to the lidocaine itself. For this reason and because lidocaine is a relatively safe and very effective anesthetic for almost all types of skin surgery, I have used it almost exclusively for skin surgery. For long or extensive procedures, a longer-lasting anesthetic such as bupivacaine (Marcaine) may be preferred. For in-depth discussion of local anesthetics, the reader is referred to deJong's (1977) excellent text. The following discussion is limited to the use of lidocaine.

Lidocaine is perhaps the most widely used local anesthetic for skin surgery today. It is usually administered as a 1 or 2 per cent solution. Some physicians are unaware that it is also available as a 0.5 per cent concentration that is completely effective for infiltration anesthesia. I have performed full-thickness scalp excision for scalp reduction procedures with 0.5 per cent lidocaine with 1:200,000 epinephrine. The patient experienced no pain at any time during the one-hour procedure. The 0.5 per cent concentration is especially helpful if a large area is being infiltrated (e.g., hair transplantation or complete infiltration for dermabrasion), thus approaching the maximum recommended dosage.

Solutions may usually be obtained either plain or with epinephrine 1:100,000 or 1:200,000. Epinephrine provides for a greatly increased effective anesthesia time, because vasoconstriction by epinephrine delays absorption from the area. This also allows for a greater maximum dosage, since anesthetic is released into the systemic circulation at a slower rate.

Epinephrine does a very effective job of curtailing small vessel bleeding during skin surgery, an advantage many surgeons would not want to do without. There is, however, the definite cardiovascular effect of tachycardia (and possible tachyarrhythmias), high blood pressure, and their possible sequelae. Despite the small dosage (as compared with the standard 0.4 cc 1:1,000 given subcutaneously for allergic reactions, etc.), side effects do occur. Interaction of propranolol (Inderal) and epinephrine may result in very serious side effects, including severe hypotension and bradycardia. Since propranolol is very widely used in both old and young for a variety of reasons (e.g., hypertension, angina, migraine headache, etc.), the surgeon should be well aware of these effects.

One study (Crabb, 1979) showed that a concentration of epinephrine as low as 1:500,000 was just as effective as higher concentrations in controlling bleeding. Since this concentration is not commercially available, the surgeon may simply dilute a 1 per cent 1:200,000 concentration with an equal amount of saline or water to make a 0.5 per cent 1:400,000 solution.

It is frequently heard that one must wait about 5 to 10 minutes for local infiltration anesthesia to take effect. If the anesthetic is partially or completely infiltrated into the deep dermis, however, the anesthetic effect is virtually immediate. Dermal infiltration will almost invariably assure a 100 per cent painless procedure. Subcutaneous injection alone is not as completely reliable in blocking all superficial cutaneous nerves. This is because of the inability of subcutaneous tissue to keep the anesthetic fluid localized as well as the dermal collagen. The disadvantage of skin surface distortion with wheal formation is usually overcome by proper incision lines drawn before infiltration. Manual skin massage can also minimize distortion in the wheal.

INFILTRATION METHOD

Infiltration is the most commonly used method of anesthetizing the operative site for skin surgery. To minimize infiltration pain, some physicians have advocated warming of the anesthetic, but I have found this to be of little benefit. Proper vibration while injecting the needle is also said to decrease the pain of injection. This may be similar to the technique used by acupuncture experts. It somehow seems a bit exotic for routine skin surgery.

The skin is entered with a 30-gauge needle at about a 30 degree angle (Fig. 3–5). Usually the needle must be advanced about 0.5 cm at

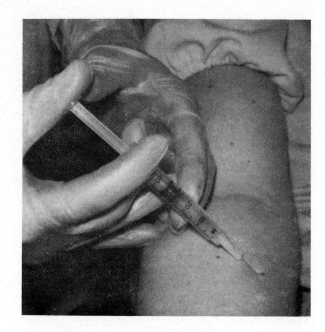

FIGURE 3–5. The anesthetizing needle enters the skin at an angle of about 30 degrees.

this angle before it enters subcutaneous tissue, although the depth varies considerably with location and skin type. Complete infiltration into subcutaneous tissue rather than dermis will have three disadvantages: (1) The time of effective anesthesia will be shorter. (2) There will be a time lag after injection before anesthesia takes effect, and anesthesia sometimes will be less than 100 per cent. (3) The volume of anesthetic used will be greater. An advantage in some circumstances is the absence of distortion of skin surface markings and topography. If lines for excision are already drawn, distortion may not be significant. When lesions such as a small pedunculated nevus or skin tags are to be removed, however, infiltration into the dermis may enlarge the lesion to several times its original size if the anesthetic infiltrates the lesion itself. This may hinder the use of the smallest circular punch or other device to excise the lesion with the shortest possible scar.

Partial infiltration into the deep dermis will cause a wheal that will clearly identify the infiltrated areas. The added tissue turgor may also be advantageous with hair transplantation and dermabrasion. Although anesthesia is almost immediate when the dermis is infiltrated, the resulting swelling may induce a transient painful sensation for a fraction of a second.

Anesthesia by local infiltration for excision of cysts and malignant lesions should be done along the lines drawn for excision. The needle usually should not enter the cyst or malignancy. Fluid injected into the cyst may enlarge it unnecessarily. For small cysts, however, a slightly larger size may be advantageous for clear identification. The pressure of additional fluid may extrude characteristic keratinous material, assuring a previously questionable diagnosis. Infiltration into a malignancy would carry the theoretical risk of spreading tumor cells beyond their present location, although practically this is unlikely with skin cancer such as basal cell carcinoma.

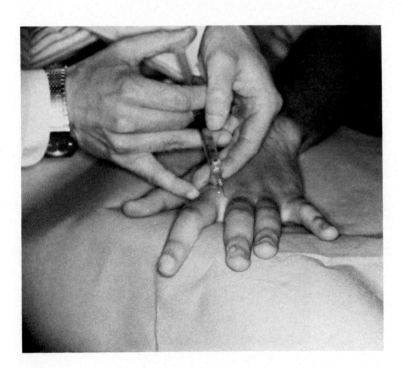

FIGURE 3–6. Injecting plain lidocaine into a web space for nerve block anesthesia of a digit.

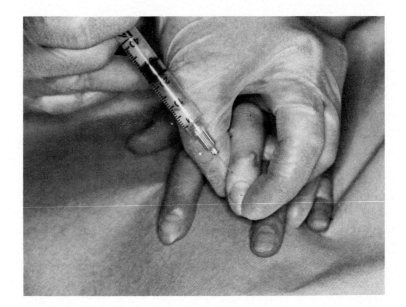

FIGURE 3–7. Infiltration of the periungual area for nail surgery.

NERVE BLOCK

Nerve block is a less frequently used but quite effective method of anesthesia for surgery. When lidocaine is used, a 2 per cent concentration is preferred for nerve block.

The most practical use for nerve block in skin surgery is for anesthetizing digits. Infiltration along the path of digital nerves in the

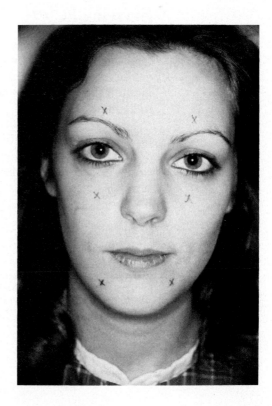

FIGURE 3–8. Locations for nerve block anesthesia of submental, infraorbital, and supraorbital-supratrochlear nerves. Note that a slightly medial injection may catch both the supraorbital and supratrochlear nerves in the same injection.

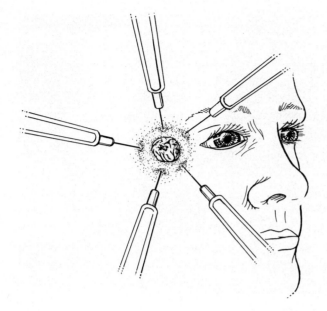

FIGURE 3–9. Field block anesthesia in a fence-like configuration around the lesion.

web space (Fig. 3–6) accomplishes complete anesthesia. For nail surgery this block is best done in conjunction with local infiltration of the periungual area after digital nerve block is performed (Fig. 3–7).

For most facial skin lesions, direct infiltration is most appropriate. For large lesions or dermabrasion, however, nerve block is a useful adjunct. Infiltration around submental, infraorbital, and supraorbital nerves is quite helpful (Fig. 3–8).

FIELD BLOCK

Field block anesthesia involves blocking of cutaneous nerves entering the area to be excised. Anesthetic is infiltrated in a fence-like configuration around a central area (Fig. 3–9). For skin surgery, this method is most useful when attempting to avoid direct injection into a malignancy (e.g., basal cell carcinoma, melanoma excisional biopsy).

If it is almost certain that the tumor does not penetrate subcutaneous tissue (e.g., small basal cell carcinoma), the needle may enter the dermis from outside the lesion. One may then proceed to subcutaneous tissue underneath the malignancy without actually injecting through the tumor itself.

REFERENCES

Crabb, W. C.: A concentration of 1:500,000 epinephrine in a local anesthetic solution is sufficient to provide excellent hemostasis. Plast. Reconstr. Surg., 68:834, 1979.
deJong, R. H.: Local Anesthetics, 2nd ed. Springfield, IL, Charles C Thomas, 1977.
Foster, C. A., and Aston, S. J.: Propranolol-epinephrine interaction: A potential disaster. Plast. Reconstr. Surg., 72:74–78, 1983.

chapter 4

SCAR
FORMATION

Any incision in the skin initiates a complex interrelated series of events that results in a healed wound. If the incision extends into the dermis, collagen formation will leave a permanent scar. Understanding the process, however, allows the surgeon to minimize the size of the scar.

WOUND HEALING

Wound healing can be separated into four stages: vascular, epithelial, dermal, and maturational. Although the stages are intimately related and overlap, the somewhat arbitrary division does help one understand the healing process.

VASCULAR STAGE

Following injury, the first response in the skin is vascular, resulting in vasoconstriction followed by vasodilatation. That allows diapedesis of the leukocytes through the basement membrane of the dilated vessel into the extracellular space, where they phagocytose bacteria and debris. Simultaneously, there is platelet agglutination at the damaged endothelium of the cut vessel, forming a thrombus that then develops into a fibrin mesh. The mesh contracts, forming a trellis that guides the capillary buds, fibroblasts, and epithelium across the wound.

EPITHELIAL STAGE

There are two substances produced by the epidermal cells that are important to wound healing. Chalones, found in the cytoplasm of mature epithelial cells, may control the mitosis of the cells. The other substance is collagenase, which fragments collagen. This latter substance probably plays an important role in preventing dermal overgrowth when a scar is forming. A question has been raised as to the role of collagenase in keloid formation, but there are no answers as yet.

In normal skin there are low levels of mitotic activity in the basilar layer of the epidermis. With injury, however, mitosis is stimulated,

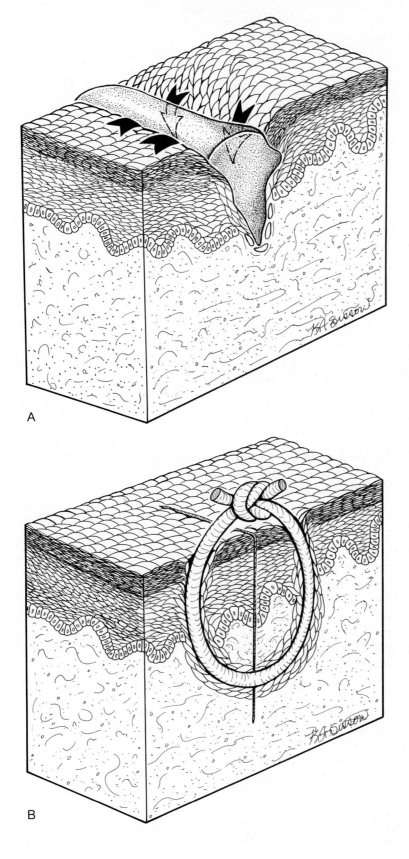

A

B

FIGURE 4–1. *A,* The earliest cellular response in the skin is found in the epidermis, which migrates across the wound surface. In a surgically closed wound, this process can epithelialize the wound surface in 72 hours. The epithelium will grow downward under a clot, here illustrated by the arrows. *B,* Epithelialization will form around a suture, leading to epithelial tunnels and cysts. Early removal of sutures prevents this. In this illustration, an external suture is illustrated. However, the tunnels also can form from a subcuticular suture when it pierces a rete peg or adnexal structure.

probably because of the loss of chalones from the mature epidermal cells. New cells are formed which grow down and across the wound surface (Fig. 4–1A). This migration of the epithelial cell occurs by extension of the cell's wall edge, which becomes a "ruffled membrane." This advances until it is in contact with another epithelial cell, at which time the cell will move in another direction until the entire structure is surrounded by other epithelial cells. Migration can close a clean incised wound in several days; however, it provides little tensile strength. This migration explains the presence of the epithelial tunnels that may form around sutures, especially in sebaceous areas of the face (Fig. 4–1B).

DERMAL STAGE

The dermal stage of wound healing involves the formation of collagen. That is divided into two phases: intracellular and extracellular (Fig. 4–2). The intracellular phase begins in the nucleus of the fibroblast, which sends messenger RNA into the cytoplasm. The RNA combines with amino acids to form protocollagen. The process requires ascorbic acid, iron ketoglutarate, protein, and oxygen and may be blocked by the protocollagen which, when hydroxylated, is excreted through the cellular membrane as trophocollagen. In the extracellular phase, trophocollagen crosslinks with its neighbor, and it is this crosslinkage that gives tensile strength to a wound. Crosslinkage may be interfered with by beta

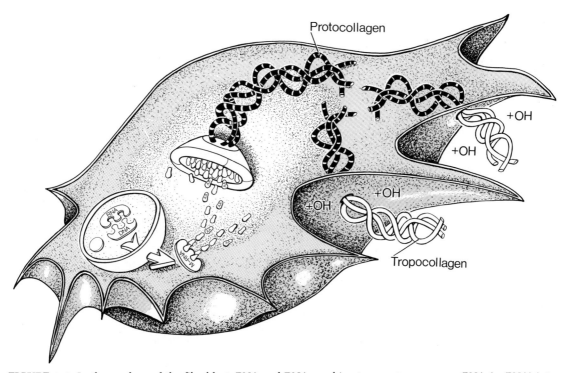

FIGURE 4–2. In the nucleus of the fibroblast, RNA and DNA combine to excrete messenger RNA (m-RNA) into the cytoplasm. This acts as a template for amino acids (AA) to begin the synthesis of protocollagen, which, when hydroxylated, is excreted through the cell wall as tropocollagen. It is this structure, when cross-linked in the extracellular space, that forms collagen and gives a wound its strength.

aminopropylnitrile (BAPN) or penicillamine. This substance was discovered in a very interesting way: A flock of turkeys was dying prematurely, especially if frightened into flight. Autopsy of these fowl revealed rupture of the abdominal aorta, and further investigation revealed that they had been eating chick peas that were rich in BAPN. BAPN had prevented the crosslinkage of the new collagen in the media of the aorta (there is a constant turnover), leading to rupture.

The appearance of collagen, viewed from the perspective of the electronmicroscope, has been shown to be like a continuous coiled ball of yarn that can be stretched to a certain extent, but beyond a limit it ruptures. Maximum tensile strength is reached about 49 days after the wound occurs and increases only slightly thereafter.

MATURATIONAL STAGE (WOUND REMODELING)

As collagen contracts, water is squeezed out of the extracellular space, which then becomes denser. Cell population diminishes, and many vascular channels are eliminated. When this occurs, the scar lightens in color and softens in consistency, losing its red or vascular appearance. In the final maturation phase, there is a balance between the production of collagen by the fibroblasts and the degradation of collagen by the epidermal collagenase. This process usually is completed after about six months but may take longer in some individuals, especially the young. Clinically this explains why application of mild pressure to a scar for about six months may help keep it flat, as by that time activity within the scar has markedly diminished. Once a scar is mature, it will not raise unless the line of initial excision, discussed in Chapter 8, is such that a hypertrophic scar could form. A true keloid, on the other hand, will continue to grow despite adequate pressure or the proper direction of the incision. The difference between these two scars will be discussed in more detail later in this chapter.

WOUND CONTRACTURE

An unclosed square wound in an animal contracts to form a stellar shape (Fig. 4–3). This process becomes static because of back tension of the surrounding skin. There are various theories to explain this process. There appears to be a contractile force in the wound bed exerted by the myofibrils pulling the edges together. That allows some wounds to close spontaneously without surgical closure, in some instances resulting in a scar that nearly equals that following a plastic closure. A good example of this is found in some locations after Mohs' chemosurgery if the wound is allowed to close spontaneously. The same process occurs to some extent beneath a skin graft, causing contracture of the wound bed.

HYPERTROPHIC SCAR VS. KELOID

Although some investigators have identified differences between a keloid and a hypertrophic scar in the laboratory, most plastic surgeons agree that differentiation is based on clinical criteria. The surgeon requires a great deal of experience to distinguish between the two in many instances.

A true keloid is a benign growth of the dermis that will recur regardless of treatment. An example of a keloid is the nodule that may

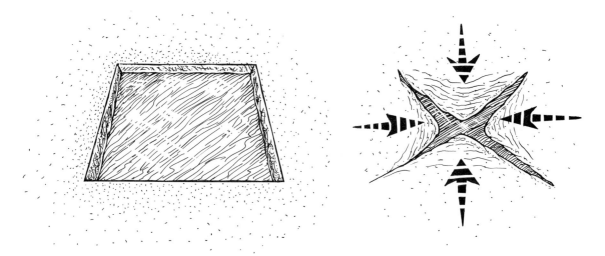

FIGURE 4–3. The process of wound contraction helps to close a wound as the forces in the wound bed pull the edges together. The contraction is limited by the tension of the surrounding tissue. Clinically, the process can be useful in closure of small wounds with loose surrounding skin. In a square wound, as illustrated, the forces of contraction (arrows) will pull the wound into the stellate shape.

develop in the area of the scar in a pierced ear. Various modalities for treatment of a keloid have been employed, including steroid injections, surgical excisions, and radiation. Keloids should not usually be completely excised because this lengthens the dermal injury and results in a larger keloid when growth recurs.

The best treatment for a keloid is an intralesional excision, purposely leaving a rim of the lesion (Fig. 4–4). This prevents the occurrence of a larger lesion in the future, which would occur if the growth were completely excised. The use of radiation in the treatment of a benign disease is questionable but may be necessary for some selected patients with keloids. It is preferable to exhaust other methods before resorting to radiation in young individuals because of the possible late effects radiation may have on the skin. Intralesional injections of steroids reduce the symptoms of pruritis, but it is unpredictable whether they will improve the appearance of the keloid because the keloid may flatten but it will also spread and may depigment.

A hypertrophic scar, on the other hand, is caused either by an error in the direction of the initial incision or by the inherent skin tension. Skin tension is due to the stretching of the skin from growth or weight gain. Such a scar is self-limiting in size, as opposed to a keloid, which will continue to grow. Examples of "tension" hypertrophic scars are found in children when the skin envelope is under pressure as growth occurs or when there is a great deal of skin tension in certain areas of the body, for example, around the shoulders or the upper back. Tension scars are also found in overweight patients. Directional errors occur from violating the principles of elective incisions, explained later in this chapter.

A way of avoiding a hypertrophic scar that may develop from skin tension is to work with loose skin. This means either waiting for the patient to grow older or selecting a period when growth is less rapid and excising only those lesions around the shoulder or upper back when the

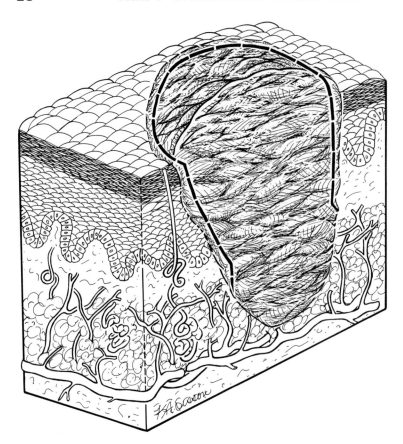

FIGURE 4–4. A true keloid is a benign dermal tumor that grows regardless of treatment. Therefore, the best treatment is to "debulk" the tumor. To accomplish this, the surgeon makes an intralesional incision, as illustrated by the dotted lines. The closure leaves some wrinkled edges, but the tumor will not be larger when it recurs because no new dermal injury has occurred.

trade-off of a large scar is worthwhile. If the hypertrophic scar is due to a directional error, changing direction through either a Z- or a W-plasty allows the scar to flatten. The stimulus for the collagen formation is removed by changing some of the scar direction into a more preferred line.

Scars with an admixture of keloid and hypertrophic elements cloud the issue, as the distinction between the two is very difficult to make. However, the distinction is very important because a directional change in a scar with a keloidal element results in a zigzag keloid. Keloidal scars are more likely to occur in individuals with increased skin pigmentation, i.e., Mediterranean, African, and Asiatic populations.

CHARACTERISTICS OF SCAR TISSUE

Scar formation is greatly influenced by the age of the patient because of two factors: the activity of the sebaceous glands and the tension of the skin. Increased sebaceous gland activity, which occurs on the face and back in young individuals, accounts for the prominent suture marks and suture tracts seen in these individuals. This is due to the rapid epithelialization from the sebaceous glands.

Increased skin tension occurs more commonly around the shoulders and lower extremities because of the "coat hanger" effect; increased skin tension may have an influence in the formation of facial scars as well under certain conditions. These may include an increase in weight or a period of growth, as this pumps up the skin, much as a balloon is filled, and causes increased skin tension in all directions. In addition, the influence of gravity causes greater tension around the shoulders and upper back. If one thinks of clothes on a hanger, it is easy to visualize the increased tension of the skin on the shoulders.

Regional variations in thickness of the skin influence scar formation. Thin skin has less dermis and rarely develops a poor scar. This author has seen a keloid in a circumcision, although that is extremely rare, but has never yet seen a keloid in an eyelid incision. Usually thin-skinned areas heal remarkably well. On thicker skin, such as that on the back and shoulder, however, there is more collagen formation. That, along with the tension factors discussed above, explains why those areas may experience the worst scars.

Heredity is also an important factor, as large scars run in some families. Although blond Caucasians may occasionally have such scars, darker skin generally has greater scar potential.

TYPE OF WOUND CLOSURE

Primary closure of a wound causes less scarring because there is less fibroblast activity and hence less collagen formation in the wound bed. Allowing the wound to heal by secondary intention under most circumstances results in more scar. There are exceptions; in Mohs' chemosurgery minimal scar potential has been achieved in some individuals. This occurs because most of the excisions have occurred in older patients with a decreasing tension in the skin envelope, less sebaceous activity, and thinning skin.

ELECTIVE INCISIONS

LANGER'S LINES

Much has been written about Karl Langer's experiments in the early nineteenth century. His drawings depicting the results of his studies became known as Langer's lines and were interpreted as elective lines of incision. This is not the case; they describe one aspect of inherent skin tension. What Langer accomplished in his experiments was to show that if an ice pick was used to produce wounds on a fresh cadaver, oval rather than round holes resulted. Those oval configurations changed directions in various parts of the body. That indicated inherent skin tension in certain areas. Curiously enough, the lines in some locations correspond to what later was described as privileged anatomic areas, such as the sternum and the dorsum of the fingers. However, Langer's experiments did not take into account the direction of the underlying muscle pull, which probably explains why following the lines does not prevent hypertrophic scars in the majority of locations. Langer's lines are of interest to the surgeon employing flap tissue, and help explain the unequal spread of a wound in such a situation. However, for the purpose of this discussion the lines are of historical interest only.

DIRECTION OF INCISIONS

The direction of the incision is the single most important factor in providing an optimal scar anywhere in the body. The age and weight of the patient, location of the wound on the body, and condition of the skin are important, but the direction of the incision is paramount.

A list of diagrams for any regional location could be memorized; however, understanding three basic principles allows the surgeon to make an incision anywhere in the body with full confidence that the least obvious scar has been provided for that individual at that particular time. The criteria are (1) placing the incision at right angles to the direction of muscle pull; (2) allowing the scar to bend; and (3) using certain privileged anatomic areas.

Right-Angle Incision

Placing the incision at right angles to the direction of muscle pull is the most important criterion in scar placement (Fig. 4–5). A scar contracts in all directions. Since there is more collagen in the length of the scar than in the width, the major contraction is lengthwise. This inhibits the stretch of the skin in that direction. A scar parallel to the underlying muscle limits the full excursion of that muscle. For example, if there is an incision lengthwise in the palmar surface of a finger, a hypertrophic scar results. As the scar contracts, it shortens, yet the extensor mechanism, as it straightens the finger, exerts a pull on the

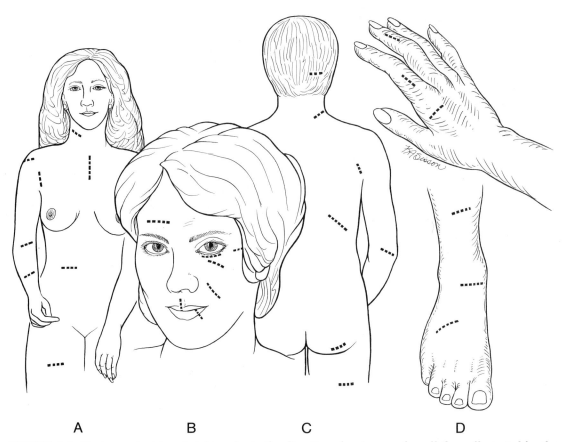

A   B   C   D

FIGURE 4–5. Placing an incision at right angles to the direction of major muscle pull (here illustrated by the dotted lines) causes the least scarring. A longitudinal incision works in some areas, such as over the dorsum of the toe (D). An incision parallel to the rim of the eye is effective (B), even though the incision is not at right angles to direction of muscle pull.

lengthwise scar. In order to prevent a rupture of the scar, the body responds by increasing the amount of collagen formation, resulting in a raised scar. If the incision is made transversely, such an effect does not occur, since no excursion of the scar is required as the muscles contract. A right-angle direction to the pull of the muscle happens to correspond to the skin creases. In some young individuals, the creases are not readily apparent, but knowledge of the underlying anatomy allows the surgeon to design a scar in the proper direction.

There are exceptions: On the dorsum of the finger, crossing one joint does not produce a hypertrophic scar in spite of the flexor pull, but crossing two joints may. On the forehead, lacerations in a vertical direction rarely give hypertrophic scarring, even though they parallel the frontalis muscle pull. This may be because the skin of the forehead is relatively thin and the bone provides a rigid surface pressing against the scar.

Bending the Scar

Allowing the scar to bend is the second most important criterion for proper direction of the scar. It is particularly useful around joints in the body or in those locations around rims of structures such as nasal alae, the eyelid, the ear, the mouth, and the mandible. Because scars contract more effectively from end to end, they tend to bowstring in areas of the body that curve sharply. This gives a notching effect, which can be prevented by putting a small Z, W, or stair step in the excision so that the scar has a spring to it and contraction does not cause a depression (Fig. 4–6A).

A scar can also be bent by placing it in the long axis of the joint. One can see by flexing or extending one's finger that the scar would bend but not lengthen or contract (Fig. 4–6B). It is the attempt of the antagonistic muscle to lengthen a scar that results in increased collagen formation, giving a hypertrophic scar.

Bending a scar is also useful around such joints as the knee and the elbow. In an area where an incision in the long axis of a joint is not possible, one can cross the joint in a zigzag fashion, allowing spring to the scar (Fig. 4–6C). An extension of this concept leads to the technique of "haptoplasty," in which an irregular lesion is excised by skimming the edges, preserving normal tissue.

Anatomic Areas

The third and final criterion for elective incisions is the use of certain privileged anatomic areas that heal without hypertrophic scars. In some areas these happen to correspond to Langer's lines; for instance, on the sternum, in the areola, and on the dorsum of the fingers and toes. The direction of the incision around the scalp and brow areas is another example of the use of a privileged area, since hypertrophic scars are rarely seen there. Scars in and around the ear and genitalia, no matter what the direction, rarely give a problem, as the skin is quite thin. In rhytidectomy, following the curvature of the ear and coming in and out of the scalp in various directions rarely results in a large scar.

ANGLE OF INCISION

Normally, in the hairless skin an incision is made at right angles to the skin surface. This allows the best and most accurate approximation

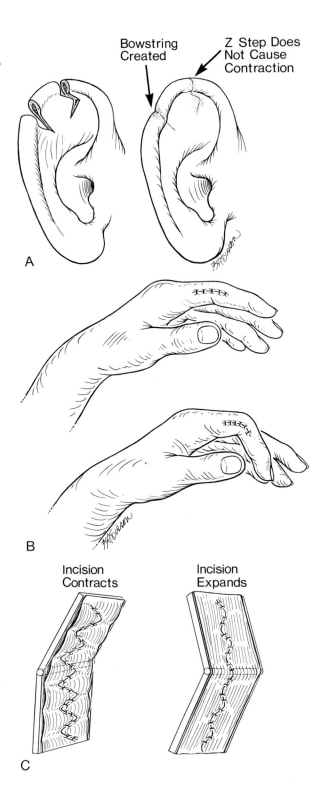

FIGURE 4–6. *A,* Because a scar contracts on its long axis, it "clefts" or forms a depression when curving around a bend (lower excision, left). Fashioning the scar so that it "bends" prevents that. Formation of an L-shaped step (upper excision) has bent the scar, preventing the bowstring. *B,* Another way to "bend" a scar is to place the line along the long axis of a joint. In this way, as illustrated on the side of the finger, the scar bends as in a hinge action and hence does not lengthen and shorten. *C,* If a scar will have to lengthen and shorten, it should be provided with a bend such as a Z or W configuration. This will allow the scar to bend and prevents the stimulation that would cause excessive collagen deposition, resulting in a hypertrophic scar. As this "hinge" moves, the Z scar can expand.

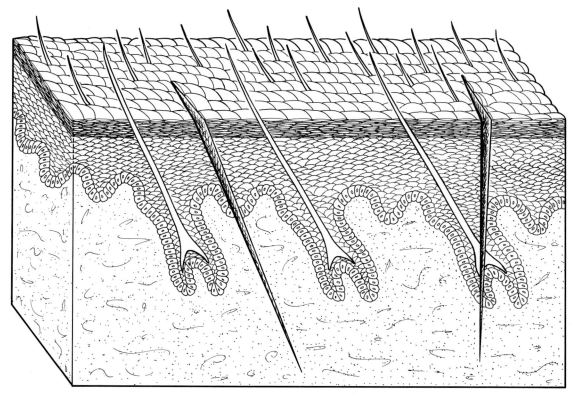

FIGURE 4–7. Ordinarily, an incision is made at right angles to the skin surface, but in the scalp this would kill some hair roots (right). By angling the blade, the surgeon preserves the follicles in those areas (left), thus avoiding an area of alopecia alongside the scar.

of the wound. A severely beveled incision, on the other hand, contracts enough that a cleft may form. In hairbearing areas, incisions must be made parallel to the hair shafts so as to preserve the hair roots (Fig. 4–7). Frequently, a large scar in the scalp is really a scar plus an adjacent area of alopecia on one side because of the loss of the hair roots. This is why one bevels the incision when taking a plug of hair for a graft. An incision in the eyebrow or on the cheeks of very heavily bearded men should also be beveled.

TYPE OF INCISION

Fusiform

For a simple incision, a fusiform incision using a 3:1 or 4:1 ratio is required for an excisional lesion. That is, if the diameter of the lesion is 1 cm, the length of that incision will be 3 to 4 cm, to prevent redundant tissue or what is called "dog ears" at the ends of the excision (Fig. 4–8). The surgeon discards significant triangles of normal skin in exchange for a smooth scar. In patients with a great deal of elasticity in the skin a shorter incision, that is, a 3:1 ratio, is usually sufficient. Older individuals whose skin has lost elasticity require longer incisions because the extra skin will not take up the slack.

"Dog Ears"

If, after the surgeon excises a wound in the fusiform manner, there is a little irregularity of the ends, the redundancy can easily be trimmed

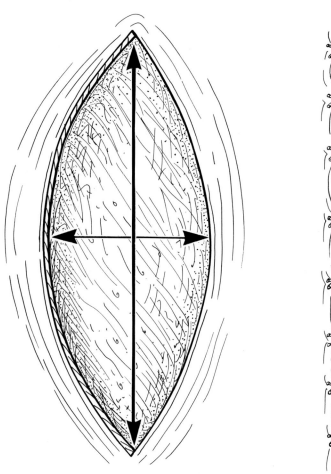

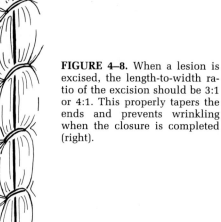

FIGURE 4–8. When a lesion is excised, the length-to-width ratio of the excision should be 3:1 or 4:1. This properly tapers the ends and prevents wrinkling when the closure is completed (right).

by lengthening the incision, overlapping the redundancy, and trimming it (Fig. 4–9). Generally, when the surgeon has gained experience, an incision can be planned so that the skin is excised without "dog ears" being formed.

Haptoplasty

A haptoplasty, or skimming the lesion and fitting the irregular pieces together, preserves as much normal skin as possible. Closure of the wound provides an irregular line, which prevents contraction of the scar as well as making the scar appear shorter to the eye. If the scar crosses some skin lines in the wrong direction it does not form a contraction because of its zigzag direction (Fig. 4–10).

Circular

V-Y Closure. In regular lesions, it is possible to effect a circular excision. Instead of excising the small triangles as one would in a fusiform incision, the surgeon can advance them to the center to form a V-Y closure (Fig. 4–11A). At first, this would seem to lead to considerably more scarring; however, the procedure transfers the loose tissue that would normally be discarded if a fusiform incision had been used into the tight center of the wound. The technique is particularly useful in the

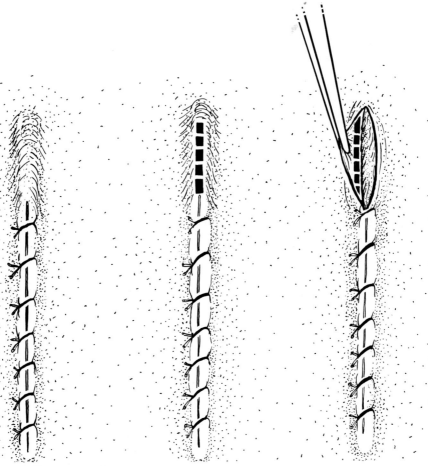

FIGURE 4–9. Occasionally, in spite of the most meticulous preoperative planning, a wrinkle or "dog ear" occurs at the end of the incision (left). This is trimmed by extending the incision (dotted line, center), overlapping the skin, and trimming the excess (right).

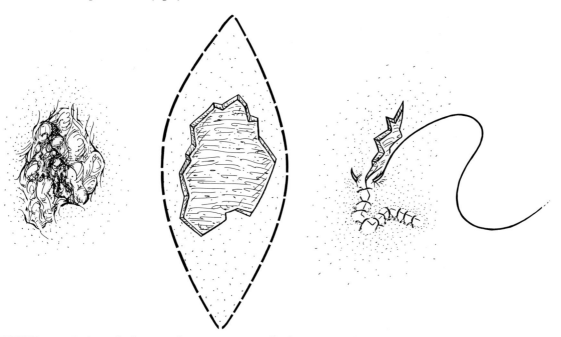

FIGURE 4–10. In irregular lesions, the surgeon can make the incision shorter than the usual fusiform incision (dotted line) by skimming the edges of the lesions and fitting the pieces together. Even though some "dog ears" must be trimmed, the resultant scar will be not only shorter but also broken in line, thus appearing shorter to the eye.

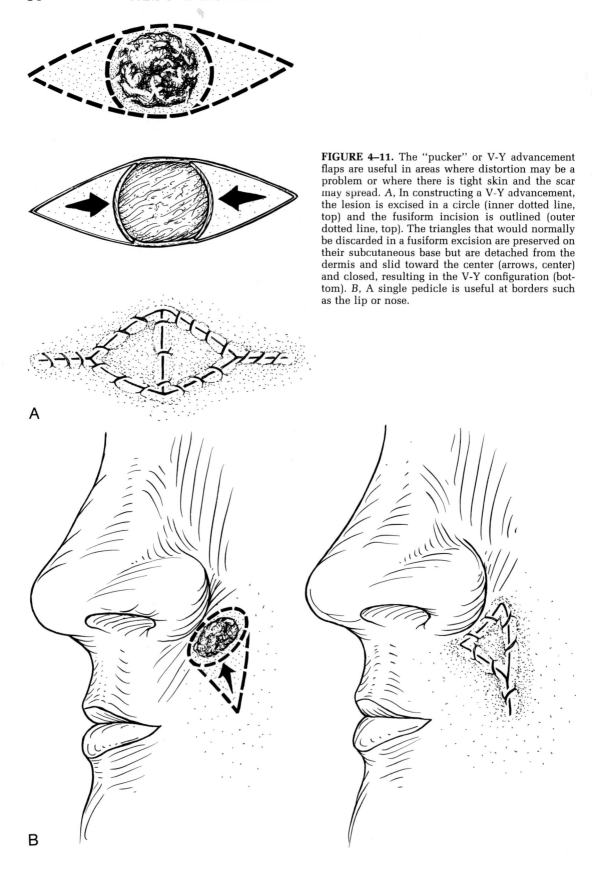

FIGURE 4–11. The "pucker" or V-Y advancement flaps are useful in areas where distortion may be a problem or where there is tight skin and the scar may spread. *A,* In constructing a V-Y advancement, the lesion is excised in a circle (inner dotted line, top) and the fusiform incision is outlined (outer dotted line, top). The triangles that would normally be discarded in a fusiform excision are preserved on their subcutaneous base but are detached from the dermis and slid toward the center (arrows, center) and closed, resulting in the V-Y configuration (bottom). *B,* A single pedicle is useful at borders such as the lip or nose.

A

B

face, the upper extremities, and the shoulder areas. Single pedicles are useful in the borders of anatomic structures such as the lip and nose (Fig. 4–11B).

A V-Y closure, like a haptoplasty, preserves as much tissue as possible and hence reduces tension in the closure and so prevents distortion of certain structures, such as the brow. In the face and upper trunk, the areas are vascular enough that the pedicles are very reliable. It can be used on the upper extremity as well, but care must be taken on the lower extremity because of the reduced blood supply.

Secondary Intention

This procedure relies upon granulation, epithelialization, and wound bed contracture. Some remarkable results have been achieved because of the pulling together of the slack surrounding tissue. Generally, as a plastic surgeon, this author prefers to close most wounds, reducing the amount of fibrosis and the chances for infection.

chapter 5

WOUND CLOSURE

TENSION

The key to a good wound closure is to avoid tension on the wound edges. The statement that "the wound gets infected" may be misleading, as in most instances what has actually occurred is that the wound was drawn together too tightly, thus reducing the blood supply at the edges and inhibiting the body's own defenses against infection. Not only do tight sutures cause this phenomenon, but rough handling of the wound, such as crushing the wound edges with heavy forceps or pressure from retractors, also contributes. The simplest way to close a wound is direct undermining, detaching the skin from the underlying fascia and allowing it to advance forward. Preoperatively, the surgeon can estimate the laxity of the skin by pinching it to see if the skin slides together easily in the region of the proposed excision (Fig. 5–1). If not, tissue should be added, and the simplest way to provide extra tissue is by adding a graft of skin.

Systemic factors influence how much tension can be safely placed on the wound; generally, however, pressure greater than 30 mm Hg on any wound causes delayed healing due to interference with the capillary blood flow. The vascularity of the area is extremely important, as the surgeon can exert a slightly greater tension on areas of the face and upper trunk than on the lower extremities, which have a poor blood supply. Tissue pressures equaling the mean arterial pressure stop skin circulation completely and would, therefore, cause skin necrosis. The age of the patient is important, as greater tension of the skin edges will be tolerated in children.

METHODS OF WOUND CLOSURE

FLAPS

Only simple advancement flaps will be discussed in this book. These involve undercutting or undermining of the skin to allow it to slide forward (Fig. 5–2). Areas of the scalp can be more difficult to close without tension because of the rigidity of the galea and the convexity of

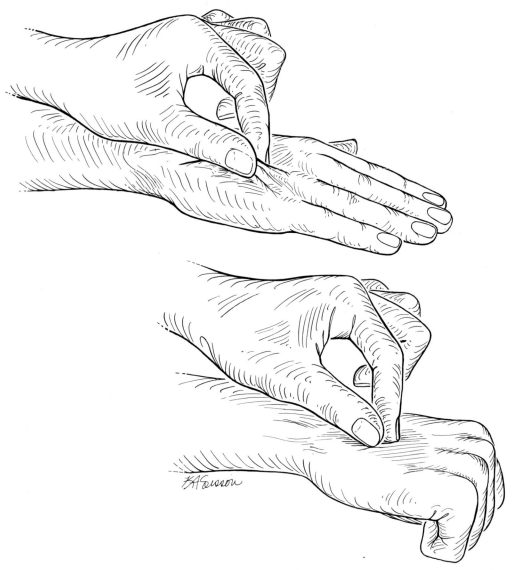

FIGURE 5–1. In the preoperative examination, pinching the skin together is a useful method for estimating the feasibility of direct closure of the skin (top). In mobile areas, it is particularly important to test the skin in *all* positions, as illustrated here in the hand. In the flexed hand, there is considerably less excess skin on the dorsum (bottom).

the skull. When one pinches the scalp together, one finds it is relatively unyielding, yet the same force applied on the abdomen brings together greater areas for primary closure. One area requires caution: On the hand the available skin changes dramatically, depending upon whether the joint is in flexion or extension. The skin on the dorsum of the hand, for example, should be tested with the fingers both flexed and extended to estimate how much skin is available for excision, as demonstrated in Figure 5–1.

GRAFTS

The simplest way to close a wound if there is insufficient tissue is by adding skin. This will close the wound rapidly; later revisions can be undertaken to minimize the scar.

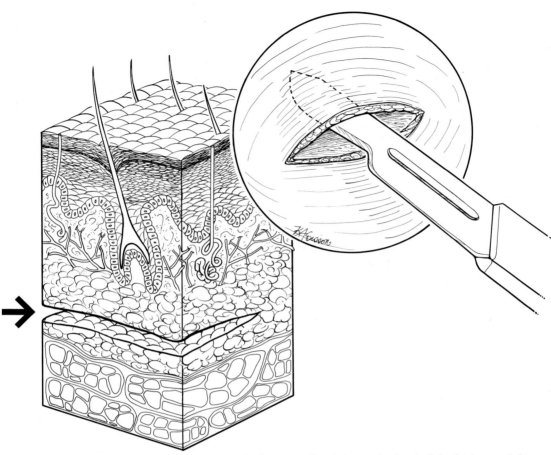

FIGURE 5–2. If the skin is tight after excision of a lesion, undermining at the level of the fat (arrow, left) cuts the fascial attachments between the dermis and the fascia. This procedure, which can be accomplished with a blade or scissors (right, inset), allows the skin to advance for closure.

Either split- or full-thickness grafts of skin may be used (Fig. 5–3). Split grafts can be taken freehand with a blade from the thenar eminence, scalp, hip, or thigh. In areas of the face where good color match is required, a full-thickness graft of skin taken from the back of the ear is very helpful, especially for use in the region of the inner canthus, the eyelid, or the dorsum of the nose. A scar will be left at the donor site, but the scar is more pronounced when a split-thickness skin graft is utilized.

A graft survives by inosculation or plasmotic circulation for up to 72 hours (Fig. 5–4). Then it becomes dependent upon vascular integrity, which results from a direct hook-up from the wound bed to the existing vessels of the graft. Anything that interferes with the revascularization process may result in the loss of the graft. Most often, this is due to hematoma formation, which separates the graft from the wound bed. A light pressure dressing on the graft for a week helps to maintain contact. In the lower extremities, because of higher hydrostatic pressures, it is advisable to maintain the pressure for several months until the graft is firmly glued to the wound bed and cannot be separated by "bulla" formation. Such pressure is best maintained by an elastic dressing or an Unna boot.

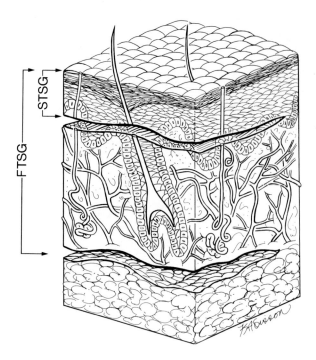

FIGURE 5–3. A graft of split skin (STSG) is taken at the level of the dermis, which allows the donor site to re-epithelialize from the remaining epithelial elements. A graft of full-thickness skin (FTSG) includes all the layers of the dermis and is taken at the level of the fat. In that case, the donor site requires closure.

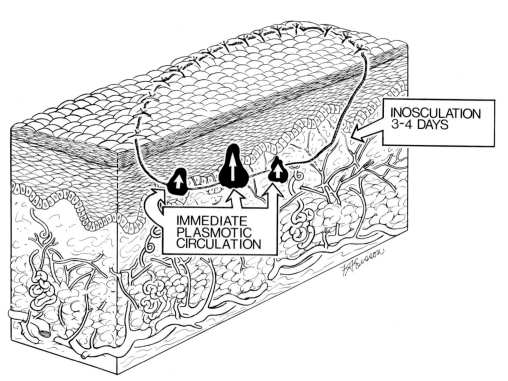

FIGURE 5–4. Initially, a graft of skin is avascular and must survive by inosculation, here represented by the arrows, until the vascular hook-up occurs on the third or fourth day.

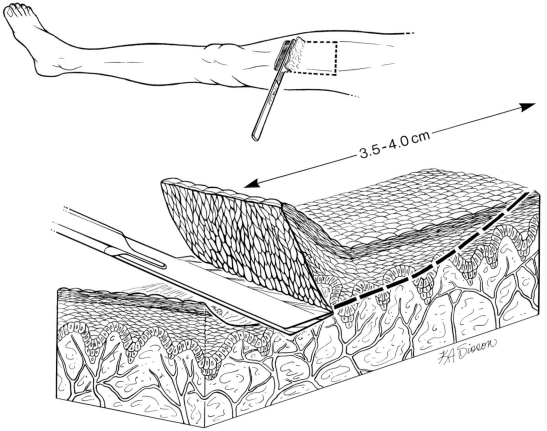

FIGURE 5–5. A small graft of split-thickness skin can be taken with a blade. A convenient location for the donor site is the anterior aspect of the thigh. On other locations, such as the buttock or lower abdomen, the donor site scar will be less noticeable. However, these latter areas are more difficult to use.

As a split-thickness graft removes the upper dermis, the wound bed heals from the residual rete pegs and skin appendages (Fig. 5–5). This is useful for larger wounds, as the donor sites heal themselves. The sites are usually treated by a gauze impregnated with Xeroform or scarlet red. Epithelialization will occur and the gauze will fall off. However, there are noticeable scars at the donor sites, which should, therefore, be selected from areas that will be hidden as much as possible.

A full-thickness graft, on the other hand, is limited in size because the donor site will not heal spontaneously and therefore requires closure, which usually results in a linear scar. This can be hidden behind the ear, the eyelid, or the groin with good results (Fig. 5–6). A full-thickness skin graft provides better skin, as all of the elements of skin are transplanted. It is more supple, causes less contraction, and provides a better color match if the skin is taken from the same general region. It is the preferred coverage for aesthetic purposes, especially on the face.

Composite grafts are grafts of more than one tissue. These are generally limited to 1 cm in size because of vascular problems encountered in larger amounts of tissue. The color match is usually excellent. A good donor site is the ear or preauricular skin in older patients. That skin is particularly useful in the thicker areas of skin such as the nasal tip, where a full-thickness graft of skin would leave a depression.

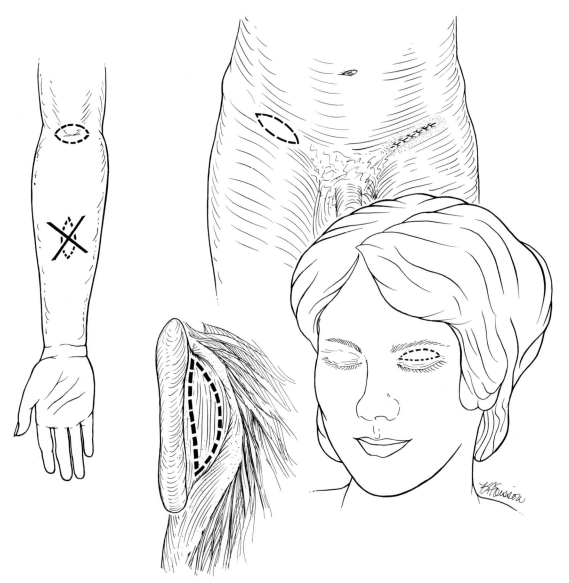

FIGURE 5–6. Excellent donor sites for full-thickness skin grafts for use on the face are the eyelid or behind the ear (right, center) because of the color match. Other useful areas are the groin and the crease of the elbow (left, top), although the color does not match as well in the face. Because a vertical incision on the forearm will leave a prominent scar, a scar should not be placed in this direction (left).

SUTURE TECHNIQUES

INSTRUMENTS AND EQUIPMENT

Excessive injury to cells provides a culture medium for bacteria. It is possible to prevent such injury by the careful use of small instruments (see Chapter 1). The best wound closure is effected with accurate approximation of all layers. Good lighting and comfortable position for the patient and the surgeon are of paramount importance in achieving this goal. For most wounds, a simple one-layered closure is sufficient. In areas of increased tension, several layers may be required if there is fascia or thick dermis into which to put a deeper layer of sutures. Fat contains very little fibrous tissue and so will not hold sutures for more than a few hours. Sutures are used to draw the wound edges together, but in the long run it is collagen formation that provides the "glue" to hold the edges together permanently. Therefore the concept of permanent sutures holding tissue together is not valid.

Properly managed, a suture should not leave an external mark. Basically, if sutures have to be left more than three or four days, a buried stitch should be used. Leaving an external stitch longer than that period of time will result in the formation of cross-hatching and/or epithelial tunnels around the suture. In practice, for the face the surgeon should use interrupted or continuous synthetic material for wound closure. As there is very little tension, these sutures can be removed in three or four days and tapes applied. For the trunk and extremities, where sutures must be left longer, it is advisable to use a buried subcuticular absorbable suture with adhesive strips on the surface (Fig. 5–7). These can be left until they have dissolved on their own. There are variations, however. In a young patient with acne, external sutures will form a mark in 12 to 24 hours because of the hyperactive sebaceous glands. In an older patient similar sutures can be left for five days with little likelihood of a problem.

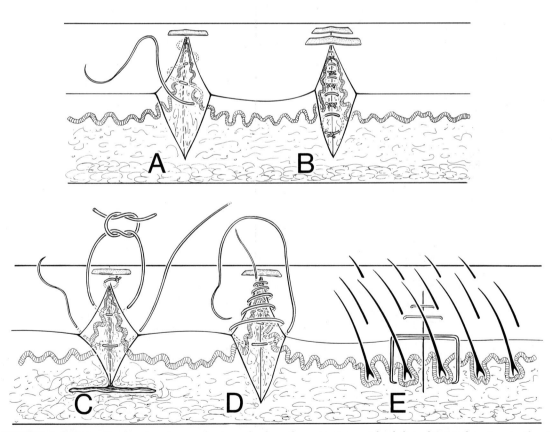

FIGURE 5–7. Subcuticular closures are best used when the sutures must be left in longer than two to three days. As illustrated in A and B, the suture may be either interrupted or continuous. In either instance, a tape (or "butterfly") completes the closure. Simple interrupted sutures are the most versatile and give the best control of the wound edges (C). In areas of thin skin, such as the eyelid, a running surface suture is effective. Taping the ends instead of tying a knot makes the removal easier (D). Staples are excellent in the scalp but leave marks elsewhere (E).

Suture marks do not form on mucosal and palmar surfaces or on the scalp when there is adequate hair.

TYPE OF SUTURE

The type of suture is less important than the principles of its use. If sutures are tied too tightly, they cut through the skin, enlarging the tunnel and forming a small scar at right angles to the incision, the so-called cross-hatch.

The sutures should be placed at right angles to the skin so that the parallelogram of forces causes eversion of the skin edges. Placing a suture too shallowly will form an inversion of the skin edge (Fig. 5–8). If the surgeon ties knots individually, there will be better control over the approximation of the wound surface, but this procedure is more time-consuming both in placing the suture and in removing it. An external continuous suture is very useful on thin-skinned patients—for instance, on the eyelid or periauricular area—where approximation of the dermis is less important. These external sutures should be of synthetic material to evoke less reaction. A continuous stitch is easier to remove, as a cut in the center allows a pull on each end to remove the entire stitch. With individual sutures swelling may bury the knot, and then the suture can be very difficult to remove, particularly in children.

A subcuticular suture is placed in the dermis under the skin and may remain. A synthetic absorbable suture rarely causes a long-term problem. A permanent nonabsorbable suture is not as useful, as it

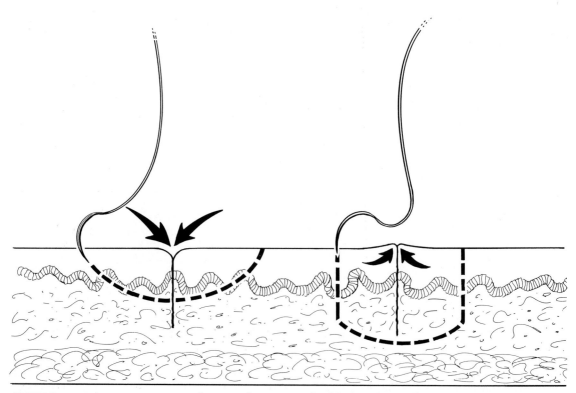

FIGURE 5–8. When using an external suture, the surgeon should place the needle at right angles to the skin surface so as to gather the deep tissue, allowing the wound to evert (dotted lines, right). If a shallow bite is taken (left), the resultant parallelogram of force will cause inversion of the wound.

eventually loses its effectiveness and may become visible or palpable. The subcuticular suture stays in for some weeks to months before dissolving, providing good tensile strength. As it will not leave any external suture marks, it is most useful in the extremities or trunk, where sutures must be left for two or three weeks. The subcuticular suture is also advisable for children, as taking their sutures out can be a major effort. The knots should be buried so that they do not come through the wound surface, as may occasionally happen.

SUTURE MATERIAL

The type of suture material is not important. The direction of the incision and closing the wound without tension have the major influence on the scar. In practice, as explained above, an absorbable material, such as a woven synthetic, is preferable for subcuticular sutures. A monofilament synthetic, which is nonabsorbable, is best for external sutures because it slides out easily on removal.

Staples are excellent for skin approximation, since they evidence low tissue reaction. They are used extensively on the hair-bearing scalp. Use in other areas may cause permanent scars from the puncture wounds. Generally, for small wounds, regular sutures are preferable.

DRESSINGS AND POSTOPERATIVE CARE

The purpose of a dressing is to support the wound edges, to reduce motion by splinting the area, and to provide some pressure to the maturing scar to keep it flat. In addition, the appearance of the wound in the patient's eyes is important. The ends of the tapes for dressings should always be cut and matched and not torn, in order to present a tidy appearance. A dressing should be easy to change and comfortable to wear and should offer no potential for harm. Casts, elastic wraps, aluminum nasal splints, and circumferential dressings around an extremity have, after swelling has occurred, led to pressure necrosis. The best dressing for a sutured wound is a strip of sterile paper adhesive tape over the surface, and at right angles to the wound to hold the edges together. A small piece of gauze placed over the strips absorbs any drainage. The gauze can be changed as needed and is fairly neat in appearance. Occasionally, a splint can be used to immobilize a joint, but rarely is a circumferential cast applied.

Postoperative care is mainly a matter of common sense. Reducing activity and keeping the wound dry for the first few days are helpful. After 24 to 48 hours, it will do no harm for the wound to get wet but it should not be soaked. This means that a patient who has had surgery to the scalp may shampoo the hair after a few days but should not soak the scalp for any prolonged period.

Antibiotics are of no proven benefit on a prophylactic basis. If a wound becomes slightly inflamed postoperatively, warm compresses by themselves will usually clear the problem. If the infection seems unusually severe or is spreading, then an antibiotic is indicated. Some patients with cardiac disease, such as Barlow's syndrome (prolapsed mitral valve) or rheumatic valvular disease, do require prophylactic antibiotics in the perioperative period. The antibiotics are usually given so that a good blood level is obtained prior to the incision and maintained during the procedure. The antibiotics are discontinued after 12 to 24 hours.

Sutures, if external, are removed from the face on the second to fourth postoperative day; tapes are applied for another week. The patient should then be asked to wear a strip of tape to apply pressure on the scar for at least part of the day or at night for another six months. If a patient adheres to this regimen, the result will be the thinnest and flattest possible scar, regardless of the area of the body.

For a patient with subcuticular sutures, the wound is checked in a week and redressed with tapes for an additional week. The patient may get the wound wet, that is, take baths, after the first week but should be asked to wear tape intermittently on the scar for six months. The patient should be asked to call if any problems develop or if the scar does not appear satisfactory. Sunlight must be avoided until the scar is mature. The patient can cover the scar with clothes, sun block, or adhesive skin tape.

SUMMARY

1. Excessive tension must be avoided in wound closure; otherwise the wound becomes devascularized and eventually infected.

2. Preoperative evaluation permits an estimation of how much skin is available for closure. This can be done by a pinch test.

3. The simplest wound closures are done by advancement flaps. If the area is too tight or there is a shortage of tissue, a simple graft can be added.

4. External sutures in the face are removed in two to four days. In areas where healing is slower and/or tension is increased, subcuticular sutures are preferred.

5. A proper dressing is both functional and aesthetic; it should offer no harm.

6. Intermittent taping of a wound for up to six months results in the thinnest and flattest scar.

PART 2

Skin Surgery Techniques Without the Scalpel

chapter **6**

THE DERMAL PUNCH FOR SKIN BIOPSY AND SMALL EXCISIONS

A special, readily available diagnostic surgical tool is the skin biopsy. No organ has been studied under the microscope at different stages of pathologic processes for so long and so extensively as the skin. The ease and negligible morbidity of the skin biopsy has allowed the accumulation of a wealth of histologic criteria to diagnose a broad range of benign and malignant skin lesions.

The skin biopsy should be used whenever malignancy is suspected, a clinical diagnosis is not absolute, or a diagnosed lesion does not behave clinically as expected. A skin biopsy should usually not be done to obtain a diagnosis the physician was not entertaining in his differential diagnosis at the time of biopsy. The surgical technique used, the depth and width of the specimen taken, the preferred location, the number of specimens needed, transportation, and special handling procedures all require at least some anticipation of the diagnosis. If the physician has no idea at all what he is going to biopsy, he may never get an accurate diagnosis. Even if the biopsy is properly obtained, in many circumstances the histologic features must be properly correlated with accurate clinical criteria. If there is any question concerning the proper biopsy procedure for a specific lesion, a textbook of dermatology or dermatohistopathology may be consulted.[1, 2] For the many benign and malignant lesions discussed in other chapters of this book, proper surgical technique has been discussed. The following is a discussion of general technique and the important variables involved in skin biopsy. Examples illustrate why such variables are important.

GENERAL TECHNIQUE

The area to be biopsied is thoroughly cleansed with isopropyl alcohol or povidone-iodine. Alcohol is preferred for most biopsies to avoid coloring clinical borders. The area to be biopsied should be marked or circled with methylene blue or gentian violet, since subsequent infiltration of anesthetic frequently distorts clinical markers (especially erythematous areas).

Plain lidocaine 0.5 to 1.0 per cent is sufficient for total anesthesia if infiltrated directly into or surrounding the area to be biopsied. For nerve block anesthesia (usually not necessary), a 2 per cent solution may be used. Lidocaine with epinephrine, 1:100,000 or 1:200,000, may be used if hemostasis is expected to be a problem, but it is usually unnecessary.

For those rare individuals allergic to lidocaine, a topical freezing spray (freon or ethyl chloride), diphenhydramine (Benadryl) infiltration, or even normal saline infiltration may be used. Some of these patients may actually be allergic to the preservative for the lidocaine rather than to the anesthetic itself. Freezing tissue with a carbon dioxide stick or liquid nitrogen is also effective, especially before quick curettage biopsy (Fig. 6–1).

The use of small needles (30- or 27-gauge) and slow infiltration minimize pain and burning sensation during injection. Some have advocated warming the anesthetic before injection to minimize burning, but this is rather ineffective and probably unnecessary.

The most commonly used instrument for skin biopsy is the skin punch. A nondisposable (e.g., Keye's punch) or disposable (Baker's) punch of sizes 2 to 6 mm or more diameter may be used. For biopsies larger than 6 mm diameter, the resulting circular or oval defect usually cannot be sutured without a prominent "dog ear" type effect. Smaller biopsies (e.g., 4 mm) may be converted to oval or elliptical defects in many areas (e.g., cheek) by stretching the skin with the thumb and index finger while taking the biopsy. The fingers should stretch the skin outward from the area to be biopsied, perpendicular to wrinkle lines (Fig. 6–2). This will result in an oval defect with the long axis parallel

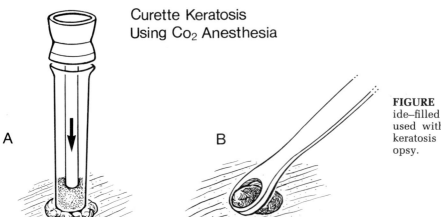

Curette Keratosis
Using CO_2 Anesthesia

A

B

FIGURE 6–1. A carbon dioxide–filled tubular applicator is used with pressure to freeze a keratosis before curettage biopsy.

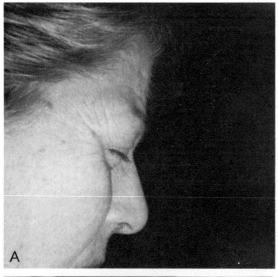

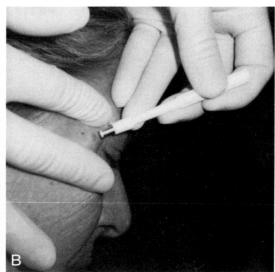

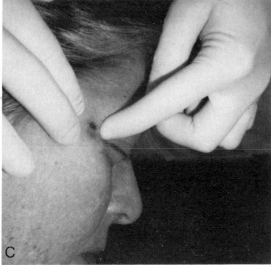

FIGURE 6–2. *A,* Nevus to be biopsied lateral to the eye. Note horizontal wrinkle lines. *B,* Four-millimeter punch biopsy to be done while stretching skin perpendicular to wrinkle lines with fingers. *C,* Resulting oval defect, which can easily be sutured without dog ears.

to wrinkle lines. It also helps to maintain hemostasis during the procedure.

Most skin lesions grow in a radial fashion, so that they approach a circular configuration in many cases. This makes the circular punch a convenient instrument for routine excision of small lesions, where the use of different scalpel blades may be a bit cumbersome.

There are two distinct advantages to using a circular excision rather than an elliptical one for small lesions with round configurations. The farther the excision extends from the border of the lesion longitudinally (forming an elliptical or fusiform shape), the longer the scar will be. The circular excision (most easily done with a circular punch) leaves a scar no longer than the diameter of the lesion. The disadvantage of a dog-ear deformity is rarely encountered or is of little esthetic significance when small lesions are excised in this fashion. In the rare circumstance of any esthetic defect after circular excision, repair may easily be done. The reverse cannot be accomplished. A long scar cannot be easily converted to a shorter straight-line scar as obtained with the circular excision. The option of such correction of circular excisions is routinely offered to patients before a punch type circular excision. This option has not been considered necessary yet by the patient or physician.

A less important advantage is the ability of the circular excision to indicate true lines of tension. This is useful only in areas that seem neutral or questionable with respect to the direction of tension of the skin.

In this circumstance the circular punch cuts through the skin without the operator pulling adjacent skin in any direction. A small oval will usually result, indicating the true direction of skin tension for that wound. One report illustrates the frequent deviation of such true tension lines from those that may be expected (Stegman, 1980). Drawings of the direction in which the oval formed with facial punch excisions illustrate this interesting point.

Punches should be extremely sharp, allowing only one circular rotation to penetrate through subcutaneous tissue. This will allow the operator to grab the specimen with a small tissue forceps, needle, or skin hook and expose subcutaneous tissue by pulling the specimen firmly and gently outward. A sharp iris scissors or scalpel should cut through the subcutaneous tissue to remove the specimen (Fig. 6–3). The biopsy site may be closed with 5-0 or 6-0 nonabsorbable suture (e.g., nylon) for skin or absorbable suture for mucous membrane. An atraumatic ⅜ circle fine point ("plastic" type) needle is suggested for the best cosmetic results. Ethicon's new "PC" needles are sharper and sturdier than their older "P" series needles. PC needles are not reverse cutting and do not seem to require this feature for smooth passage through tissue. Even a 4-mm biopsy is best closed with two sutures to minimize the dog-ear effect that may result with one central suture (Fig. 6–4). With a 5-mm biopsy the two sutures may be placed one third the diameter from each end.

In some areas a butterfly bandage for small biopsies may suffice,

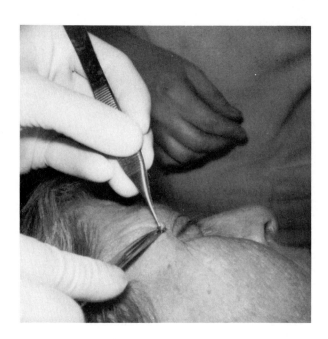

FIGURE 6–3. Adson tissue forceps pulling specimen up and outward. Tips of fine iris scissors cutting subcutaneous tissue to release specimen.

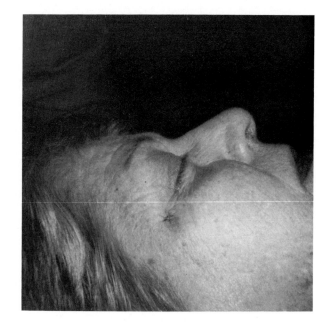

FIGURE 6–4. Closure of 4-mm punch biopsy with two 6–0 nylon sutures without dog-ear effect.

but it is not as reliable as suturing. Without suturing the patient must be more careful not to get the area wet postoperatively. Sutures are usually removed on the face in three to five days and on the trunk in approximately seven days.

Another method of treating the biopsy defect has been to cauterize or electrodesiccate. This usually shrinks the area to about one half its original size, filling the defect with dead, necrotic debris. Alternatively, it may be filled with Gelfoam or similar material and covered. In most patients this will heal adequately in two to three weeks, but healing is less predictable than with suturing.

In a short, unpublished study I compared suture closure with electrodesiccation or butterfly closure. Biopsies were on the same normal skin area in the same patient, since they were done to evaluate long-term effects of psoralen and ultraviolet light (PUVA) in the treatment of psoriasis. Pus or drainage, inflammation, and prolonged healing time were all more prominent in the nonsutured areas. Cosmetic results were superior with suturing.

One argument against suturing small biopsies is the sterile set-up and assistance necessary to make suturing the small defect truly an aseptic procedure. Many patients (e.g., leukemics, severe diabetics, etc.) require such aseptic suturing technique to avoid the hazard of an open wound prone to infection. Such an aseptic technique may be performed routinely in the hospital and office as follows:

1. Thoroughly prepare the area widely with povidone-iodine or alcohol and let set for at least two minutes. The unsterile hand or glove, however, will never touch the prepared area. If the operator is to be free to perform the procedure alone and to avoid the necessity of sterilizing everything from the anesthetic bottle to the specimen bottle, his hands will not be able to be "sterile."

2.   Instruments are taken from a sterile surface (e.g., an autoclaved paper or sterile towel pack) permitting only their handles to be touched with the unsterile hand. When the instruments are not being used, their sterile working ends are returned to the open sterile paper or towel.

3.   If sponging is necessary, sterile gauze is taken from the sterile biopsy pack or separate sterile wrapping. It is grasped at the ends and sponging is done only with the sterile center (Fig. 6–5A).

4.   Suture packs may be opened without touching the sterile needle. The needle may be grasped with a sterile needle holder (Fig. 6–5B). The suture is pulled out only a few inches and the outer suture pack is held with the other unsterile hand. The suture is passed through the entire wound and the needle holder grasps the needle as it exits from the opposite side (Fig. 6–5C). The suture is then pulled through and out of the pack to avoid dragging the suture on unprepped skin. When the end of the suture is about one inch from the entrance site, the opposite side is cut, with several inches remaining for easy instrument tying (Fig. 6–5D).

5.   If a second suture is needed, the free end of the suture is grasped with the unsterile hand (this end will not pass through the skin) and the needle end is allowed to hang freely. One quickly learns to grasp the needle again in the proper position while it is hanging freely (Fig. 6–5E). Twisting the suture held at the end by the unsterile hand can reposition the needle for easy grasping with the sterile needle holder jaws. Keeping the unsterile end taut will prevent a sagging suture from touching unprepped skin during the second passage of the suture (Fig. 6–5F). This process can be done three or four times with an 18-inch suture, allowing enough suture to use instrument tying.

6.   After all sutures are passed through the skin, they are then instrument tied. The needle holder will become "unsterile" during tying because it will grasp ends already touched by unsterile hands (not passed through prepped skin). It is therefore necessary to do all instrument tying after all the sutures have been passed through the skin. The above aseptic procedure may be performed without assistance and should take only five minutes or less to complete. Of course, a completely sterile surgical technique with assistance or all necessary items (anesthetic, etc.) sterilized is an alternative. The above method is really quite simple and completely sterile and may be used whenever circumstances require it.

Another technique for obtaining a full-thickness skin biopsy is the small diamond- or elliptical-type excision. If only a small specimen is needed, a No. 11 or Beaver-type blade is helpful. A disadvantage is that defects are usually larger than the 3 to 4 mm required in some circumstances. An advantage is the more ideal configuration of the wound, with less tendency for a dog-ear defect. There is also less tension across the wound than with a circular configuration. Of course, a complete sterile set-up as for routine excision will be necessary.

If the operator is sure that the lesion penetrates only the epidermis and superficial dermis, a biopsy may be obtained by a superficial shave with a scalpel or razor blade. He must fully anticipate the depth of the lesion and accurately shave to this depth if he wishes a complete pathologic specimen. In some instances he may want only a sample from superficial dermis and epidermis in order to leave a more acceptable cosmetic result. An example would be shaving or scissors excision of a

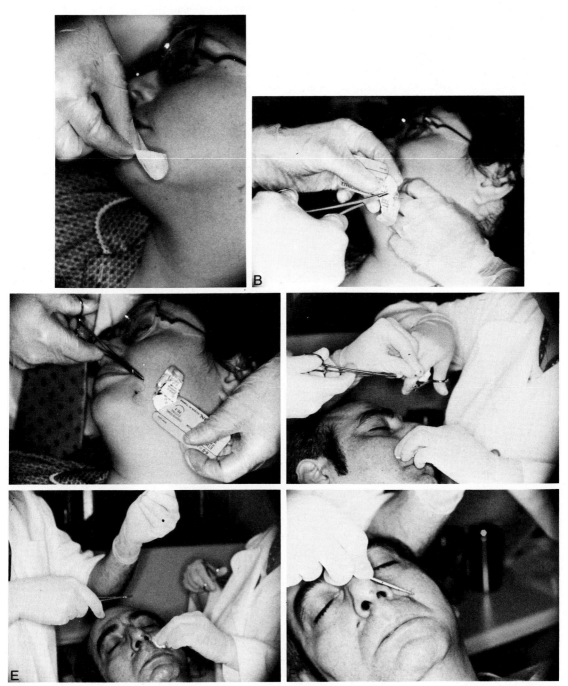

FIGURE 6–5. *A,* Sponging with sterile center of sponges. *B,* Grasping needle from suture pack with sterile jaws of needle holder rather than with fingers. *C,* Needle holder grasping the needle as it emerges on the opposite side of the wound. *D,* Cutting the suture while the needle holder is still grasping the needle. *E,* Grasping the free-hanging needle with the sterile jaws of the needle holder while the unsterile hand holds the end of the suture. *F,* Passing the needle through the skin for a second suture while holding the suture taut to prevent sagging onto surrounding undraped and unprepped skin.

pedunculated nevus from the trunk (Fig. 6–6). If one wishes to avoid a noticeable depression with a shave procedure, one should infiltrate anesthetic peripherally into the subcutaneous fat to avoid distortion of the surface by injecting into the dermis, allowing a shave parallel to the surface plane. The patient should be aware that some of the lesion may remain (Fig. 6–7), since subsequent biopsy and interpretation by an uninformed pathologist could lead to misdiagnosis (e.g., melanoma). After shave biopsy, hemostasis may be rapidly obtained by a nonstaining solution of 35 per cent aluminum chloride in 50 per cent isopropyl alcohol applied with a cotton-tipped applicator and brief pressure. Light electrodesiccation has the advantage of shrinking the defect but the disadvantage of being the classic injury (burn) for excessive scar formation in those patients so predisposed. It should be noted that if melanoma is ever suspected, biopsies to the depth of subcutaneous tissue only should be performed. This allows for a proper evaluation of tumor thickness and depth, so critical for prognosis and treatment choice for this tumor.

Skin biopsy for epidermal lesions may also be obtained effectively with a dermal curette. Effort should be made to include a sizable specimen and to avoid putting other small fragments in with the specimen. If there is suspicion that the lesion is penetrating the dermis (e.g., early squamous cell carcinoma in an actinic keratosis), a deeper punch or excision biopsy may be performed.

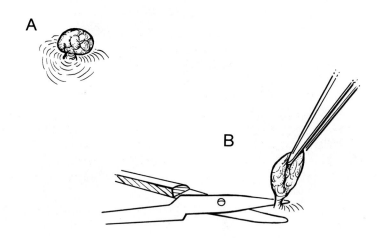

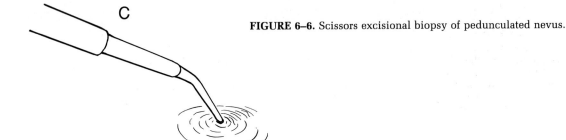

FIGURE 6–6. Scissors excisional biopsy of pedunculated nevus.

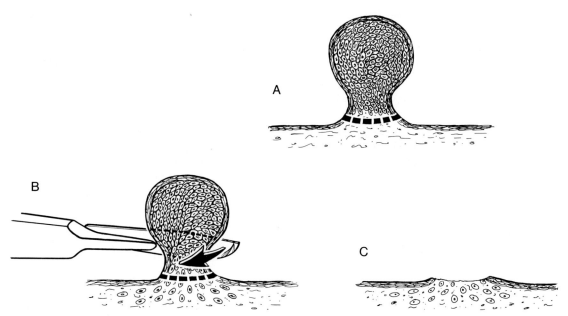

FIGURE 6–7. *A,* Pedunculated nevus with nevus cells at or above the surrounding tissue. *B,* Pedunculated nevus with some nevus cells penetrating lower into the dermis. *C,* Shave biopsy may leave nevus cells behind, depending on the level of the shave and the location of the nevus cells.

A curette specimen of a lesion may be submitted for three reasons.

1. The operator may be virtually sure of the diagnosis and proceed immediately with curettage and electrodesiccation treatment after obtaining the curette specimen (e.g., nodular basal cell carcinoma). Effort should be made to include a large single section of the tumor for biopsy with the first passing of the curette. The pathologist should be informed that this is not a complete excision specimen and, therefore, comment as to adequacy of excision of tumor in the specimen margins is inappropriate. If a punch biopsy is done prior to curettage and electrodesiccation treatment, it may invalidate this method of determining tumor margins with the curette. If the tumor is limited to the dermis, the curette may distinguish between the soft consistency of tumor tissue (with basal cell carcinoma) and the firmness of the healthy dermis. If the tumor itself or a previous biopsy has penetrated the dermis into subcutaneous fat, the curette cannot easily distinguish between tumor-involved fat and soft, healthy fat, The curette biopsy is then preferred if curettage-electrodesiccation is to be the method of treatment. I sometimes prefer excisional surgery for cutaneous malignancies because of the histologic check that can be performed on intact specimens to determine if tumor has been adequately removed. One exception is the excellent cosmetic result obtained with curettage-electrodesiccation on small primary basal cell carcinoma, especially on the nose.

2. Some surgeons will perform curettage to determine more accurately the margins of tumor before planning the excision lines (usually for basal cell carcinoma). In this circumstance a curette specimen may be obtained for biopsy, but the intact excisional specimen should also be submitted.

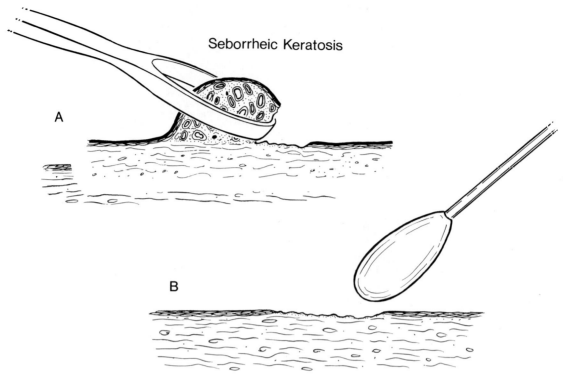

Seborrheic Keratosis

FIGURE 6–8. The curette easily removes a seborrheic keratosis with sharp shearing force. Aluminum chloride styptic is applied after removal.

3. Last, removal by curettage may give the best cosmetic results for some lesions (especially seborrheic keratoses). The typical clinical features of seborrheic keratoses and the characteristic clean separation between keratosis and underlying dermis detached by the sharp shearing force of the curette usually make biopsy unnecessary for the experienced curette operator (Fig. 6–8). In this instance the curette is a very useful instrument for rapid diagnosis.

DEPTH AND WIDTH OF SKIN BIOPSIES

Most biopsies of the skin should penetrate to subcutaneous tissue and include a good portion of subcutaneous fat if it is available. Care should be taken not to damage nerves that may run just beneath the fat (e.g., facial nerve). Strictly epidermal lesions may be biopsied by shave or curettage, as mentioned above, but the diagnosis should be firmly established to avoid the necessity to re-biopsy or submission of insufficient tissue for diagnosis. Lesions that involve the fat primarily, such as erythema nodosum, may be biopsied by excision technique to assure an adequate specimen for diagnosis. The early inflammatory process of scleroderma is seen mostly in the subcutaneous fat. Changes in the fat combined with compatible changes in the dermis will make the diagnosis easier for the pathologist in this circumstance. In a possibly related disorder, Shulman's syndrome or eosinophilic fasciitis, scleroderma-like clinical skin changes are seen; however, the primary pathology is seen in the superficial fascia in this circumstance. In diseases such as polyarteritis nodosa and dermatomyositis, the pathology of muscle may be more helpful than that of skin. In this circumstance both muscle and skin may be biopsied at the same time by surgical excision.

PREFERRED LOCATION

Although skin lesions may be seen in many different areas, a knowledge of the pathologic process may favor one location over another. A lesion of erythema nodosum would be best biopsied away from the immediate pretibial area to include a generous portion of fat. Deposits of amyloidosis may be better seen in rectal mucosa than in normal-appearing skin, although there may be deposits in both areas.

Most bullous skin lesions should be biopsied early in the development of a vesicle. Early re-epithelialization of a bulla may distort the original site of cleft formation that is critical for diagnosis of most bullous diseases. Subsequent inflammation and even infection may alter the type, intensity, and location of inflammatory cells helpful in categorizing bullous skin disease. A biopsy at the edge of an early erythematous vesicle in dermatitis herpetiformis may show the accumulation of neutrophils at the dermal papillae at the intact border and the adjacent subepidermal separation of the vesicle. A similar biopsy may show eosinophilic spongiosis at the border and suprabasilar acantholysis of the vesicle in pemphigus vulgaris. On the other hand, biopsy of skin to reveal the IgA deposits of dermatitis herpetiformis by immunofluorescence should be done on normal skin.

THE NUMBER OF SPECIMENS NEEDED

In many circumstances more than one skin biopsy specimen will be needed. Skin lesions may look clinically different, such as the varioliform and papular lesions of pityriasis lichenoides et varioliformis acuta (Mucha-Habermann disease). It may be difficult to obtain a biopsy with characteristic histologic features in a clinically borderline papulosquamous eruption (e.g., lichenoid eruption), necessitating two or more biopsies to increase chances of detecting the characteristic pathology. If a disorder persists and the first set of biopsies have shown only nonspecific changes, repeat skin biopsies may give additional information needed for diagnosis. Early lesions of mycosis fungoides may be present for years before histologic changes are characteristic enough to make a diagnosis. More well-developed infiltrated plaques in the same patient at the same point in time may prove the diagnosis of mycosis fungoides when other less-developed lesions do not. With this lymphoma of the skin or its possible precursors (e.g., parapsoriasis or poikiloderma atrophicans vasculare), multiple biopsies of different lesions should usually be done at first. If no diagnosis can be made and the lesions persist, skin biopsy should be repeated at a later date. This is particularly true if lesions increase in size, infiltration, or number.

If multiple specimens are needed for different diagnostic studies (e.g., culture, immunofluorescence, hematoxylin and eosin staining, electron microscopy), a single larger biopsy by elliptical excision may be preferable. This larger specimen may then be sectioned appropriately.

TRANSPORTATION AND SPECIAL HANDLING OF THE SPECIMEN

Specimens submitted for regular staining with hematoxylin and eosin should be put in bottles containing 10 per cent formalin or the preferred fixative of the pathologist interpreting these biopsies. The volume of fixative should be several times that of the specimen. If specimens are mailed, the volume of fixative should be sufficient to cover the specimen in all positions of the specimen bottle (e.g., on its side), and tight screw caps (not snap-on caps) should be used.

It will usually take the pathology laboratory one day or more to process a routine specimen for permanent paraffin blocking and staining. If the diagnosis is needed sooner to initiate therapy (e.g., severe bullous disease) or to guide excision with difficult tumors at surgery, a frozen section should be done. Specimens should be quickly submitted in saline-moistened gauze. Sutures or permanent dyes on the margin of tumor specimens are necessary to determine which margins, if any, may have tumor involvement.

If culture for bacteria, acid-fast bacteria, or fungi is to be done, the specimen should be submitted in a sterile container. Non-bacteriostatic water or saline may be used if some delay in transportation is expected. The laboratory will grind the specimen and plate it appropriately. They can also do smears and stains with the specimen, if requested. The physician should submit a separate specimen for paraffin sectioning with bacterial, acid-fast, and fungal stains done.

Immunofluorescent staining for detection of immunoglobulins, complement, fibrin, and various antigens (e.g., hepatitis antigen) is a vital diagnostic technique for diagnosing a broad spectrum of skin and internal disorders. Specimens should be quick frozen in liquid nitrogen and stored at −70°C until processed. Michel et al. have described a transport medium that may obviate freezing. The laboratory should be thoroughly familiar and satisfied with this medium for routine biopsies.

Electron microscopy can be quite helpful in diagnosing the malignant cells of mycosis fungoides and the site of blister formation in different varieties of epidermolysis bullosa. It may also be used to detect viral particles. Special fixatives (e.g., glutaraldehyde) and refrigeration are frequently used for such biopsies.

REFERENCES

1. Fitzpatrick, T. B., et al.: Dermatology in General Medicine, Textbook and Atlas. 2nd ed. New York, McGraw-Hill, 1979.
2. Lever, W. F., Schamburg-Lever, G.: Histopathology of the Skin. 6th ed. Philadelphia, J. B. Lippincott Company, 1983.
3. Michel, B., Milner, Y., and David, K.: Presentation of tissue-fixed immunoglobulins in skin biopsies of patients with lupus erythematosus and bullous diseases—preliminary report. Invest. Dermatol., 59:449–552, 1973.
4. Stegman, S. J.: Excisions of the face. Dermatology, 77:43–45, 1980.

chapter 7

ELECTROSURGICAL TECHNIQUES

Throughout this book there are brief mentions of the acceptability of electrosurgical techniques for various skin lesions. The authors, by training and experience, clearly prefer scalpel excision for most lesions penetrating the deep dermis or subcutaneous tissue. When strictly epidermal lesions or lesions in the very superficial dermis are approached, however, superficial destructive methods such as electrosurgery can be quite acceptable.

The well-defined primary basal cell carcinoma may also be treated with this method. For instance, lesions on the nose may require grafting if excised with the scalpel. In such a circumstance, curettage and electrodesiccation produce superior cosmetic results in most circumstances.

The following is a brief description of equipment and technique used for electrosurgery. Reference to specific lesions in subsequent chapters will comment on the acceptability of electrosurgery for that lesion.

ELECTROSURGICAL UNITS

One of the oldest and most widely used units is the Birtcher Hyfrecator. It is used for both electrodesiccation techniques and electrocoagulation. The high-frequency damped spark gap current it supplies is not meant for electrosurgical cutting techniques. I find very little need for this cutting feature in skin surgery. It may be more useful in general surgery.

The Hyfrecator is a lightweight (2-kg) unit that may easily be kept in a drawer, mounted on a wall with two screws supplied, or mounted on an optional three-caster lightweight stand. It is supplied with a standard handle and a straight needle electrode. The current is activated by a foot switch only, which is permanently attached to the unit (older models had foot switches that were connected separately). A new unit is now available with an optional switch on the handle. For monopolar use there is a high and low output connection. For bipolar use two biactive outlets at the right of the unit are used. Total output is adjusted for monopolar and bipolar use by a simple dial. The dial is turned clockwise from 0 (off) to 100. The same dial turns the unit on and off.

A large number of accessory handles and electrodes are available for this unit (see Appendix). Short and long, straight and angled electrodes may be used. Tips for electrodes may be thick, extremely fine (for epilation and small telangiectasis), blade shaped, ball shaped, looped, and double pronged (for biactive use). One available electrode accepts the metal base of a 30-gauge needle for use as an electrode itself.

An indifferent electrode plate is available and should be used when coagulating blood vessels with small hemostats. It may also be used for more direct and intense current flow. When the plate is firmly in contact with the patient's skin over its entire surface, current will flow directly through the lesion being treated to the plate and back to the machine (ground). With monopolar techniques the current may disperse diffusely depending upon the surface area and adequacy of grounding without the ground plate. The indifferent electrode grounding plate must be connected to one biactive terminal and the working electrode to the other biactive electrode (see Appendix). A new biactive coagulating forceps is available from Birtcher. The tip of the forceps grasps the vessels and the surgeon depresses a foot switch to activate current. It works quite well and eliminates the need for a ground plate or hemostat in most circumstances. The ground plate is not needed because current flows from one tip of the electrode to the other and back again. The cord has two plugs that connect to the two bipolar sockets. It is autoclavable and reusable.

The Bovie and Bantam Bovie units have the additional feature of cutting current. These are very popular units in the hospitals and may be either wall mounted or placed on portable stands. The unit may also be used with or without a grounding plate. A slight disadvantage is the manual spark gap setting that must be done before using the Bantam Bovie. The unit is also considerably heavier than the Hyfrecator. A similar wide range of electrodes is available. Like many other units that are sold to hospitals, the cost is significantly more than for the Hyfrecator. Some of the older floor models have been discontinued for more than 15 years, and parts are no longer available when the spark gap deteriorates.

For the physician who wishes a hand control unit rather than a foot switch, a relatively inexpensive unit is the Electricator (see Appendix). This may be mounted on the wall or on a small stand with an instrument tray attached. A ground plate is available; however, the connection on these can be quite loose. This allows the connection to fall out if there is any pulling on the ground plate.

Several other very fine electrosurgical units are available. The physician should compare electrodesiccation and electrocoagulation capacity (and electrosurgical cutting if needed), size and maneuverability (depending upon the surgical suite), available electrodes and accessories, the ability to use the unit with a grounding plate, and finally the cost. Before buying the unit it is helpful, if possible, to actually practice with a large piece of raw meat that is well grounded. Subsequently cutting through the treated area will reveal the depth and extent of desiccation and destruction.

Thermal cautery is less frequently used for skin surgery and is less versatile. There is no spark gap current, but a metal tip that is heated with electrical current. Superficial destruction and hemostasis may be achieved with such units.

One may obtain a permanent thermal unit with finger control (e.g., National unit) and a temperature control dial. Various disposable models are available in sterile wrapping (e.g., Concept line). I use such a battery-operated unit for penetrating a nail plate to release blood under pressure from a subungual hemorrhage. Smaller units of the same type may be used in eyelid surgery.

ELECTRODESICCATION AND FULGURATION

Technically, electrodesiccation refers to drying up tissue (desiccation) with electric current. The term is used loosely and involves varying degrees of destruction of tissue, from coagulative necrosis of protein to complete carbonization of tissue. For the same voltage output, a longer time of application, a finer needle, and a shorter distance between the electrode and tissue will all cause greater tissue destruction. With the above variables constant, greater voltage output will cause greater tissue destruction.

The term "fulguration" is frequently used interchangeably with "electrodesiccation." However, it actually refers to delivery of the electric current to tissue without direct contact of the electrode with the tissue. The term "fulgurate" (Latin: *fulguratus*—lightning) derives from the variable spark gap between the electrode and the tissue.

LIGHT ELECTRODESICCATION OF SUPERFICIAL LESIONS

Many lesions that are limited to the epidermis and superficial dermis may be eradicated with light electrodesiccation. The diagnosis should be assured or biopsy of viable tissue taken before destruction with electrodesiccation.

A fine needle set at a fairly low voltage will give more control when treating such lesions (e.g., fibroepithelial tags, small flat warts, xanthelasma). For more destruction the total time of treatment may be increased, giving more control to the operator. Although current may be quite intense with a fine needle (another reason for using low-output settings), such a needle enables the physician to treat very small portions at a time. This minimizes the effect of too much electrodesiccation in one spot. By subsequently decreasing time or output, the physician may quickly correct small errors.

1. In many circumstances a small amount of lidocaine 0.5 to 1.0 per cent is injected intradermally with a 30-gauge needle (Fig. 7–1A and B). If the lesion is close to skin color and relatively flat (e.g, flat wart), it may be colored with a marking pen or dye before anesthetic infiltration. This avoids losing the visible borders with subsequent tissue swelling and blanching due to injection. Extreme care should be taken to color the entire lesion but not more than that to avoid administration of too little or too much electrodesiccation.

2. Some patients prefer to have the procedure done without anesthetic. This is acceptable for light electrodesiccation in some circumstances. If the patient isn't sure (when treating multiple lesions), inject

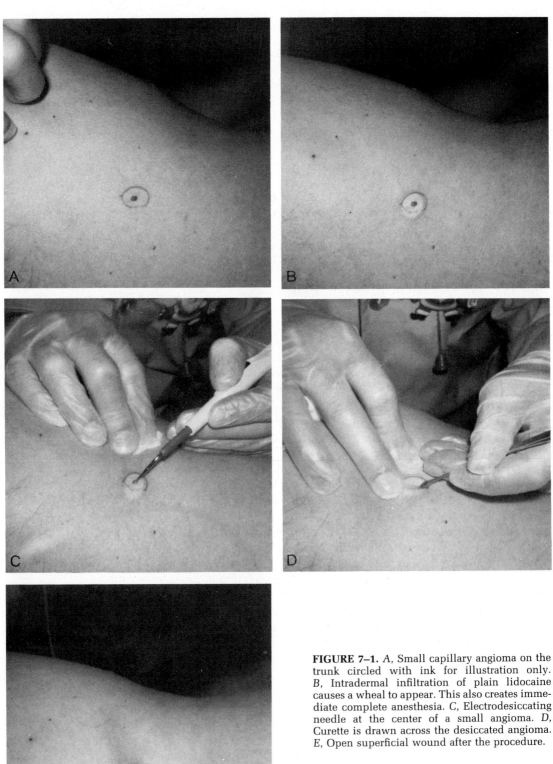

FIGURE 7–1. *A*, Small capillary angioma on the trunk circled with ink for illustration only. *B*, Intradermal infiltration of plain lidocaine causes a wheal to appear. This also creates immediate complete anesthesia. *C*, Electrodesiccating needle at the center of a small angioma. *D*, Curette is drawn across the desiccated angioma. *E*, Open superficial wound after the procedure.

anesthetic into one lesion and treat another without anesthetic. Have the patient evaluate the pain of the injection itself versus the pain of electrodesiccation without anesthesia. If the pain is about equal or less without anesthetic, the procedure may be done this way. Treatment without anesthesia (a) saves time, (b) avoids the rare possibility of allergic reactions, (c) eliminates the immediate cosmetic problem (although small) of dots of blood from multiple injections. Anesthesia must be used, however, if the patient moves to such an extent that normal skin is inadvertently electrodesiccated.

3. The electrodesiccating needle is placed directly on the lesion surface near the center (Fig. 7–1C). In this manner if too much current is being delivered or the time of application is subsequently too long, the lateral spread of tissue destruction will be less likely to involve normal tissue. This will not necessarily avoid deeper destruction, however.

4. The foot switch or handle switch is initially depressed for the shortest time possible, just enough to turn the unit on for a fraction of a second.

5. The physician then observes the adequacy (too little or too much) of tissue destruction.

6. If anesthesia is not being used, the patient response is observed. If the patient cannot tolerate the procedure without moving, anesthesia must be used. As mentioned, this avoids the possibility of contact of the electrodesiccating needle with normal skin when the patient moves.

7. The heat alone of light electrodesiccation is usually enough to cause the epidermis to separate from the dermis. After the initial electrodesiccation, therefore, a very light curettage may be done to evaluate the extent of destruction and epidermal separation. A 2- or 3-mm dermal curette (oval or circular type) is held at about a 30-degree angle from the horizontal and drawn across the treated area with light downward pressure (Fig. 7–1D). An alternative method to remove separated epidermis alone (e.g., in treating premalignant actinic keratosis with no dermal invasion), gauze may be rubbed across the treated area with slight downward pressure applied.

8. The above maneuvers will delineate the lateral extent of epidermal separation. If treatment has not been adequate at lateral borders (e.g., edges of actinic keratoses fail to lift off underlying dermis easily), additional electrodesiccation of these areas is performed.

9. The depth of destruction may be evaluated in two ways, both requiring some experience to interpret. (a) The uniform diffuse bleeding from the exposed dermis is more profuse as the depth increases. This will be seen only when slight force is used to remove the surface debris that has been electrodesiccated, exposing noncauterized dermal blood vessels. (b) When surface crust has been removed, an experienced operator can gauge the depth of destruction by the visible depression in relation to surrounding skin. Any anesthetic injected intradermally will expand the dermis significantly. This will make the depression from electrodesiccation appear deeper than it really is if compared to surrounding skin that has also been infiltrated.

These considerations are quite important when attempting to minimize subsequent under- and overcorrections for benign lesions. For premalignant lesions (e.g., actinic keratosis), the primary concern is eradication of dysplastic epidermis and even a small amount of superficial dermis if early invasion is suspected clinically. Unnecessary deep destruction, however, should be avoided if possible. Most patients with multiple facial actinic keratoses should have excellent cosmetic results from most forms of therapy (electrodesiccation, cryosurgery, topical 5-fluorouracil).

10.   Electrodesiccation is repeated if the depth or lateral extent of destruction is deemed inadequate with the first pass. Treatment again should be brief and administered with low power output. Additional electrodesiccation can always be done for undertreatment, but nothing can be done to correct overtreatment.

11.   When electrodesiccation is to be continued on a bleeding base, the prior application of an effective styptic (e.g., 35 per cent aluminum chloride in 50 per cent isopropyl alcohol) has several advantages: (a) It prevents blood from spattering. This can also be a hazard for transmission of hepatitis virus (about 1 in 1000 carriers in the United States) by contact with mucous membranes. Blood will easily reach the conjunctival surface and mouth of the physician and his assistant when spattering occurs. (b) Blood accumulates quickly on the electrodesiccating needle, decreasing its effectiveness. (c) Electrodesiccated blood on the surface of the wound decreases the effectiveness of treatment. (d) Fine control of the procedure is lost because of the poor visualization of underlying tissue and a variable degree of destruction because of interposed blood and coagulum of variable thickness.

APPLICATION OF TOPICAL STYPTIC AGENTS

A cotton-tipped applicator thoroughly saturated with aluminum chloride is applied directly to the bleeding surface with pressure for an average of 3 to 10 seconds (rarely longer application with pressure is needed). If bleeding has stopped, immediate additional pressure is applied for 1 or 2 seconds with a small piece of gauze to remove excess aluminum chloride solution. Aluminum chloride in isopropyl alcohol is very slightly irritating if left on normal skin in excess quantity. The isopropyl alcohol is flammable, so the excess should be removed before additional electrodesiccation. No danger exists, however, with the small residual left after a quick sponging with gauze to remove the excess.

Immediately after superficial electrodesiccation the wound can usually be left uncovered (Fig. 7–1E). If the patient wishes a bandage for aesthetic reasons, a simple adhesive bandage strip, a small piece of gauze, or a Telfa pad may be applied. The bandage may be removed when the patient returns home. It need not be reapplied except for aesthetic coverage during healing.

DEEP ELECTRODESICCATION

The most common lesion treated with deeper electrodesiccation is basal cell carcinoma. The techniques are similar to those previously described, with a few variations. The following uses the basal cell carcinoma as an example of a lesion treated by deep electrodesiccation.

1.   A line may be drawn with a marker completely around the lesion, staying about 3 to 5 mm from the border at all points. Surrounding tissue will contract significantly during electrodesiccation, so this line

may serve as a marker 3 to 5 mm from *visible* borders before treatment is started.

2. Infiltration anesthesia is accomplished as previously described. A field block–type infiltration is preferred here. This avoids the theoretical possibility of spreading tumor cells with infiltration through the tumor itself. Infiltration is performed in a circular fashion (Fig. 7–2A). Both subcutaneous and dermal layers are infiltrated.

3. A short waiting period for anesthesia to take effect (2 to 3 minutes) may be necessary when the tumor area itself is not directly infiltrated.

4. The first curettage should preferably be done with a sharp curette that is as wide as the tumor itself (this may, of course, be the shortest diameter of the tumor). This will allow for removal of most of the tumor body relatively intact with the first curettage, providing an excellent pathologic specimen.

5. The curette is placed firmly on normal skin about 1 mm distal to the tumor edge. It is held at an angle of approximately 30 to 40 degrees from the horizontal (Fig. 7–2B).

6. Firm downward pressure is exerted while still on normal skin.

7. The curette is slowly and firmly drawn toward the edge of the tumor.

8. At the edge of the tumor only firm downward pressure is exerted at first, until complete resistance is met.

9. At this step the curette is drawn toward the operator, maintaining constant pressure downward throughout the maneuver (Fig. 7–2C).

10. At the proximal edge of the tumor the curette is slowly brought up. Firm downward pressure is still exerted as the curette is drawn toward the operator.

11. The total specimen is placed in 10 per cent formalin for pathologic examination and confirmation of diagnosis. Pathology reports should not comment on the tumor edges or borders, since this is irrelevant for such a specimen. The laboratory slip should indicate "curette specimen for diagnosis only."

12. A styptic such as 35 per cent aluminum chloride in 50 per cent isopropyl alcohol is firmly applied to the base with a cotton-tipped applicator (as described above).

13. Whenever the applicators are lifted from the base, small gauze sponges are immediately applied with pressure in their place. This soaks up excess styptic solution and blood and achieves further hemostasis.

14. Styptic may be reapplied as many times as necessary to achieve hemostasis (Fig. 7–2D).

15. With the base now visible, curettage is again performed (*before* electrodesiccation).

16. The curette is firmly drawn around the sides and the base of the tumor. This is continued until firm dermal tissue is encountered on all borders. Tissue largely invaded by basal cell carcinoma (except the sclerosing type) will have a soft consistency.

17. A smaller dermal curette (e.g., 2 to 3 mm) is used to check all the borders for any soft spots that may indicate tumor extension.

18. A styptic is again applied to provide a visible dry field. Continual use of this styptic provides a clear field for the operator and

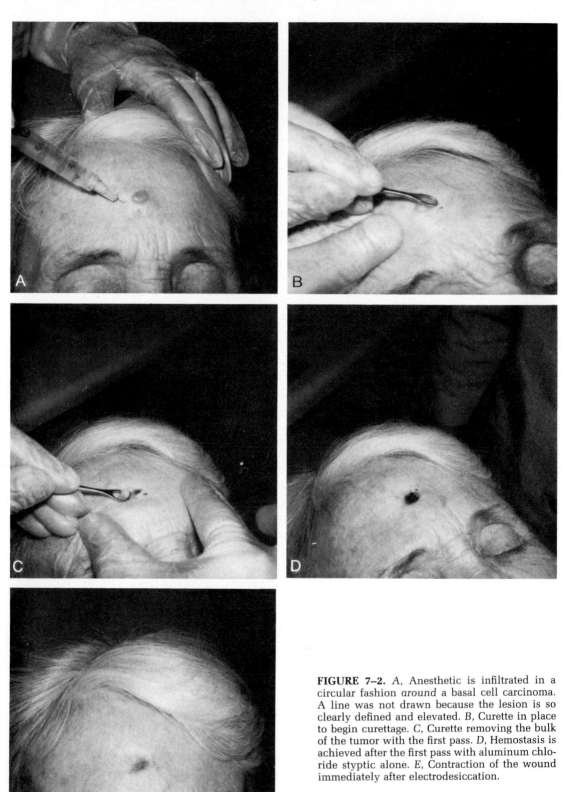

FIGURE 7–2. *A,* Anesthetic is infiltrated in a circular fashion *around* a basal cell carcinoma. A line was not drawn because the lesion is so clearly defined and elevated. *B,* Curette in place to begin curettage. *C,* Curette removing the bulk of the tumor with the first pass. *D,* Hemostasis is achieved after the first pass with aluminum chloride styptic alone. *E,* Contraction of the wound immediately after electrodesiccation.

avoids spattering of blood and coagulum accumulation on the desiccating needle.

Note that we have avoided using electrodesiccation until after thorough curettage to determine tumor borders accurately. Unlike electrodesiccation, the styptic agent will not alter the consistency of surrounding tissue. This tissue consistency is critical to the accurate perception of soft tumor tissue with the curette.

19. With a dry wound surrounded by firm dermis on all sides, the operator proceeds with electrodesiccation. A medium point needle is used with a medium to strong current setting. The operator works from the inside to the outer borders of the lesion. He will notice the contraction of tissues toward the center as he proceeds (Fig. 7–2E). The wound will contract and scar in a similar fashion during the subsequent healing process.

20. A very sharp curette is again used to remove burned tissue formed by the electrodesiccation.

21. A final electrodesiccation is performed, extending at least to the border drawn with a marking pen before the procedure was begun (Fig. 7–3A).

Note: Many operators have suggested three or more curettage and electrodesiccation steps. Electrodesiccation before thorough curettage to firm dermis may alter the soft tumor consistency used as a guideline for adequate removal with this method. When the wound is thoroughly curetted to reach firm dermis on all borders before the first electrodesiccation, multiple subsequent procedures seem unnecessary. In fact, they may penetrate healthy dermis into the subcutaneous tissue. Before electrodesiccation is performed, it is also necessary to determine if the curette will freely penetrate soft tissue (basal cell carcinoma) into the subcutaneous layer. If this happens, the curette can no longer be used to determine the tumor margins and an alternate method of removal is suggested (e.g., scalpel excision). Basal cell carcinoma penetrating subcutaneous tissue is seen in only a very small percentage of cases and may represent a more aggressive tumor subset.

The number of curettings (*before* electrodesiccation) should be determined by the presence of firm tissue on all borders with both large and small curettes. This number will vary with each tumor and, therefore, cannot be precisely defined.

I would like to mention briefly what is perhaps the most important aspect of electrosurgical or any other chosen surgical modality. Unlike studies that may randomly assign different methods of treatment for basal cell carcinoma (e.g., electrodesiccation vs. scalpel excision vs. irradiation vs. Moh's technique), the practicing physician must select his *preferred* approach for each individual lesion he sees. Experience, surgical ability, and the independence of his decisions should give the qualified physician better results than studies that may include residents in training or protocols that may restrict decision-making somewhat. *Unbiased* studies cannot and should not necessarily weigh such experience and independent selection, as they are extremely variable parameters; however, they are still clearly present and to the added advantage of many practicing physicians. To be able to select one case for Moh's technique, another for wide excision and graft, and another for electrosurgery, based upon experience and personal preference, will yield

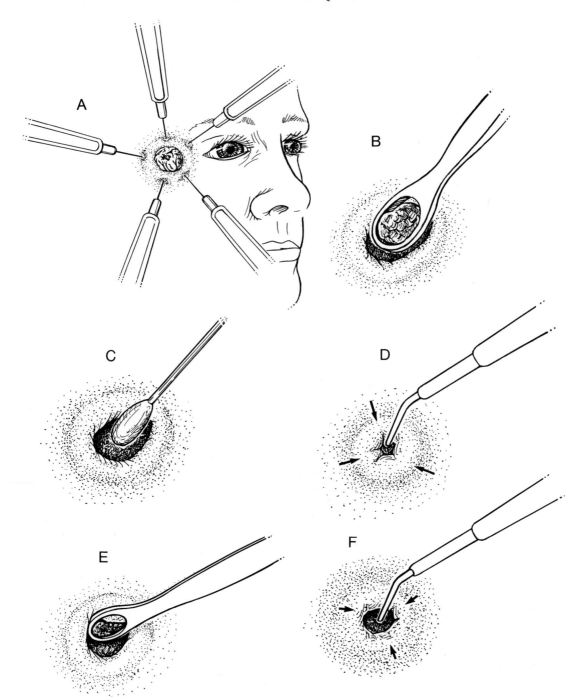

FIGURE 7–3. *A,* Field-block method of anesthesia around a basal cell carcinoma. *B,* Curettage of tumor bulk. *C,* Aluminum chloride styptic for hemostasis and clear visualization. *D,* Electrodesiccation with contraction of the wound. *E,* Removal of charred material. *F,* Final electrodesiccation.

results much better than those published in most series. To decide intelligently that superficial curettage has been adequate in one case and that penetration of the curette into subcutaneous tissue in another requires wider excision and checking of the pathology of the margins should definitely work to the experienced operator's (and patients') advantage.

PART 3

A Regional Approach to Skin Surgery

chapter 8

REGIONAL APPROACH TO EXCISIONAL BIOPSY

DIRECTION OF INCISION

A working knowledge of the principles of elective incisions allows the surgeon to minimize the scar for that particular individual at that particular time in his life regardless of its location on the body. As discussed in Chapter 4, the incision must be placed at right angles to the direction of major muscle pull, be allowed to bend (for instance, in the long axis of a joint or in a zigzag fashion), or be placed in certain privileged anatomic areas.

Elective incisions are fusiform, circular, or irregular. Fusiform excision in a 3:1 or 4:1 arc, tapering at the edges and undermining (if necessary), allows direct approximation of the edges. A circular excision of a lesion preserves the tissue that would normally be excised at the corners in a fusiform excision. Those corners are moved toward the center in V-Y fashion. This maneuver is particularly useful in areas of tight skin to reduce distortion. A haptoplasty or irregular excision skims the border of a lesion. Putting the small points together preserves normal tissue and effects a zigzag closure that is useful in certain areas.

The incision should always be at right angles to the skin surface except in areas where the hair is to be preserved, such as the brow and the scalp. There a bevel is required to preserve the hair roots.

CLOSURE

Types of closure influence the final scar. Generally, primary closure reduces scar formation and results in a thinner scar. However, Mohs' chemosurgery has shown us that closure by contracture and epithelialization (secondary intention) produces some rather remarkable results in areas of loose skin. For example, fairly large lesions in the face

75

and even of the nasal tip of older persons often heal as well as if a full-thickness graft had been used.

REGIONAL VARIABILITY

The quality of the scar varies from region to region in the body in spite of an optimal scar direction. This is because of variations in function, in blood supply, in tension, and in thickness of the skin.

The function of a region is particularly important in managing a wound, as initially rest and elevation of the part hasten wound healing. For example, it is best to elevate the leg and put it at rest. However, patients with lesions of the extremities continue to be ambulatory, which increases the healing time and the resultant scar. If there is an extensive excision, it is worthwhile to apply a good pressure dressing to reduce the swelling and to place the patient on crutches to rest the part as much as possible.

The blood supply is richest above the clavicle and least pronounced in the lower extremities, particularly around the ankle. The blood supply to all areas decreases with age and, again, this decrease is most noticeable in the lower extremities. Clinically, this means that there can be less tension in wound closures in these regions. It should be noted that in patients with systemic diseases, such as diabetes or arteriovascular disease, or localized disease, such as venous stasis, the blood supply in the lower extremities may be so poor that the mildest trauma causes an ulceration that will not heal.

AGE OF PATIENT

Young people have more internal skin tension because they have more elastic tissue and an ever-expanding internal mass of bone and muscle when growth is occurring. Since elasticity of tissue decreases with age and growth ceases in the teens, the older the patient after this point the less "inherent" skin tension is present. This explains why a child may develop a hypertrophic scar that, when revised in later life, will not become hypertrophic again. For children, there are periods of slow growth that may be seized upon for necessary excisions.

The pull of gravity places more tension in the skin over the shoulders, upper back, and chest. This explains many of the hypertrophic scars that commonly develop in those areas, although the intensity of reaction decreases with age. Therefore, unless strong clinical indications suggest otherwise, it is best to defer excisions in those areas until the patient is older.

Skin thickness influences the scar. Basically, the thinner skin has thinner dermis and therefore requires less collagen in the scar for strength. For example, the eyelid and genitalia are the areas of thinnest skin, and generally scars in these areas are not detectable without close observation. In contrast, the skin of the back, which is the thickest in the body, forms very noticeable scars.

The palm and the sole of the foot form very little scar tissue unless there is a directional error in scar placement. The apparent thickness of the skin in these areas is usually the result of a thick epidermis rather than a thick dermis.

FUNCTION

The function of the part is important. For instance, an abdomen generally has loose surrounding tissue because of its range of flexion and extension, its expansibility, particularly following pregnancy, and its predisposition to fat deposits. An area of difficulty can be the dorsum of a hand. Extension of the fingers presents a picture of loose skin, but flexion quickly makes it apparent that there is little skin to spare in those areas and caution must be used.

Generally, placing the area in functional position to use the maximum amount of skin (i.e., abdomen in extension, hand in flexion) and using the "pinch test" show how much tissue is available for excision. This is particularly useful in the face to determine if surrounding areas will be distorted after an excision.

Facial lesions easily lend themselves to closure because of the mobility of the area. Using the pinch test on the pretibial area, by contrast, shows that there is little skin mobility there. Because that area is in a lower extremity, the surgeon can ill afford a tight closure because of reduced blood supply and increased hydrostatic pressure.

REGIONAL CHOICES

HEAD AND NECK

Scalp. The scalp is not as easily closed as might appear. At first consideration it appears to be a well-vascularized mobile tissue. However, because of the rigidity of the underlying galea and the convexity of the cranium, the scalp actually has poor mobility and only small closures can be achieved.

Excisions and primary closures, even with wide undermining, are limited to less than 10 per cent of the circumference of the scalp. Incisions should be beveled to preserve hair follicles. Many "wide scars" in this area are a result of alopecia on one side of the scar from a nonbeveled incision. In addition, in the preoperative planning, the surgeon should consider the possible pattern of baldness that will occur in most men. For instance, taking a hair transplant site from the lower occipital area may result in the donor scar's showing when loss of lower hair occurs.

Electrocoagulation of vessels, even the larger arteries, such as the temporal, is usually sufficient to control bleeding in the scalp. Infection is rare. Shaving of the area makes the surgery more convenient, but it is unnecessary, as shaving does not alter the infection rate for surgery of the skin.

Sebaceous cysts in the scalp are not attached to the dermis as they are in other regions of the body and therefore do not require excision of skin. Incision of skin with an enucleation of the cyst from the subcutaneous tissue is easily achieved. Anatomic layers of the scalp are remembered by the mnemonic "scalp" (skin, subcutaneous tissue, aponeurosis (galea), loose areolar tissue, and periosteum). The vessels and nerves run in the subcutaneous tissue. Basically, in this area the anatomy is fairly risk free. The surgeon should, however, beware of the lesion fixed to the cranium, particularly near suture lines and in the midline. Although such a lesion may communicate intracranially, a radiograph may not show that communication.

Face. The tissue of the face is loose, well vascularized, and easily closed. Incisions made in the proper direction generally heal with little problem. However, the face is prone to acne. Individuals in the age group during which acne is common may have significant scarring because of the activity of the sebaceous glands. Oily skin will show wide, depressed scars as well as prominent suture marks. Dry skin heals with finer scars because of the inactivity of sebaceous glands. Infection is rarely a problem on the face.

The seventh cranial nerve is the most important structure in the region. After it emerges from the stylomastoid foramen, the nerve becomes more superficial as it travels distally. This is particularly the case after it emerges from under cover of the parotid gland, which varies tremendously in size from individual to individual (Fig. 8–1). The nerve

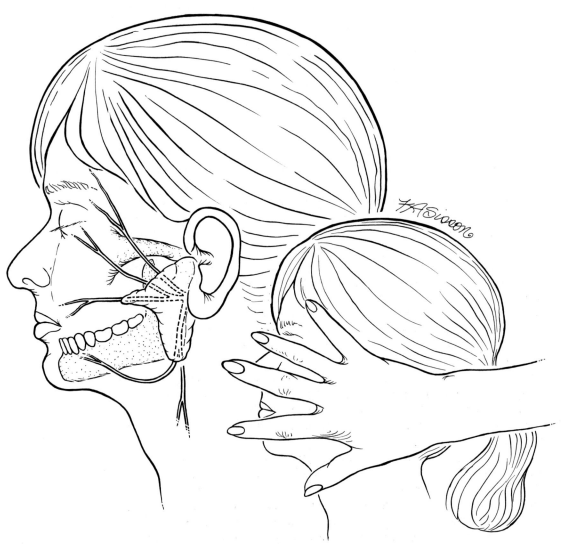

FIGURE 8–1. The seventh nerve emerges from the stylomastoid foramen, pierces the parotid gland, and innervates the facial muscles in five main branches, which become more superficial peripherally. Those branches are especially vulnerable after they leave the protection of the parotid gland. Placing the left hand on the right side of the face and the right hand on the left side of the face permits one to locate the five branches—cervical, mandibular, buccal, zygomatic, and temporal.

is particularly exposed to damage near bony prominences, such as the mandible and the zygomatic arch.

Ear. Excisions of lesions of the ear are generally limited to 4- or 5-mm closures, as beyond that, unless the underlying cartilage is excised, a full-thickness graft is needed. On the rim of the ear and in the earlobe, where bowstringing of the scar may occur, small, step-like incisions should be used for excisions if they go around a corner.

Nose. Excisions of lesions in the nose present a problem because of the tight skin, especially near the tip. Pinching the skin together enables the surgeon to estimate the size of excisions allowable, generally not more than 0.5 cm for a primary closure. Even with excisions as small as 0.5 cm, the ala may be distorted if the excision is close to it. Because of the sebaceous glands, sometimes wounds of the tip granulate in an older individual and eventually leave very little scar. Although this technique is generally frowned upon by plastic surgeons, who are more accustomed to closing wounds, it does work well in some older individuals. On the rim of the ala, if there is an incision that goes around the corner, staggering the scar with a W-plasty or L-shaped excision prevents a bowstring effect. Grafts of full-thickness skin generally cause a dent, which later "fills out" to some extent. Composite grafts from the earlobe (limited to about 1 cm) may overcome this problem. Too deep an excision may result in a nasal fistula (Fig. 8–2).

Lip. Elective incision of lesions of the lip should follow the radial pattern of the orbicularis muscle. A scar that extends over the chin, mandible, or curve of the vermilion may cause a bowstring effect. However, a small zigzag in the vermilion or a W-plasty around the curve of the mandible usually prevents this. Great care must be taken in the approximation of the white roll of the vermilion border, as a notch or misstep is not uncommon and is very noticeable (Fig. 8–3). It is often worthwhile to mark the vermilion border with a No. 30 needle and methylene blue prior to the infiltration of local anesthetic, as adrenalin blanches the tissue enough that normal anatomic landmarks are often obscured, especially under a bright light. This effect may also occur in other areas of pigment change, such as the areola in the region of the nipple.

One can normally excise up to one third of the lip in older patients and still effect a primary closure. Excisions of greater proportions usually require flap techniques. Excision of the vermilion of the lower lip for extensive leukoplakia can be closed with an advancement flap by undermining the vermilion to the buccal sulcus. The labial artery is superficial to the muscle and usually encountered. The facial nerve has branched sufficiently in the lip that isolated damage should not occur.

Eyelid. Extensive excisions of the lesions to the upper eyelid should parallel the tarsal crease, which is approximately 10 mm above the ciliary border. In most persons, 5 to 15 mm of skin of the upper lid can be excised, depending on the age of the individual. Too great an excision prevents closure of the lid, which results in lagophthalmos and a feeling of dryness of the eyes or even corneal ulcers. Ectropion after excision in the upper eyelid is very uncommon. A good preoperative test is to pinch together the estimated amount of skin to be resected and observe if the eyelid can still close.

Smaller excisions can be made in vertical fashion, but the line of

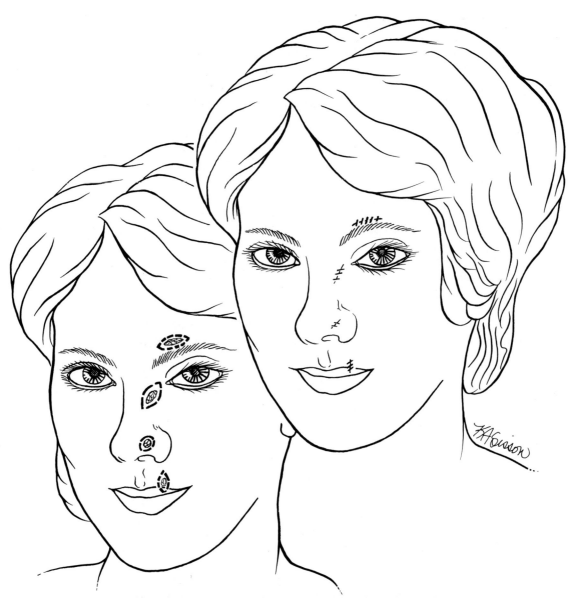

FIGURE 8–2. The surgeon should design excisions to correspond to skin creases, which can be shown in animation. When a border is involved, such as the white line of the lip, careful attention must be paid to its proper alignment. After excision of suprabrow lesions (left), closure will result in some elevation of the brow (right). Excision of lesions of the tip of the nose may require addition of tissue, such as a composite graft, because simple closure may result in distortion of the nasal ala. Subcuticular V-Y pedicles do not work well in this area. Over the bone, however, direct closure is frequently possible because of the looser skin.

excision should change as the excision goes laterally into the "crow's feet." If the patient is asked to squint, these lines will be obvious.

In the lower eyelid, smaller excisions must be made or skin added to prevent an ectropion. The closer to the ciliary border, the less skin can be removed (generally only 2 or 3 mm). The incisions should parallel the ciliary border. As the surgeon moves further away from the edge of the eyelid, larger areas can be excised. The incision should begin to slant in the radial fashion of the orbicularis oculi. Especially in an older individual, who has a lax tarsal plate and hence less support of the lower

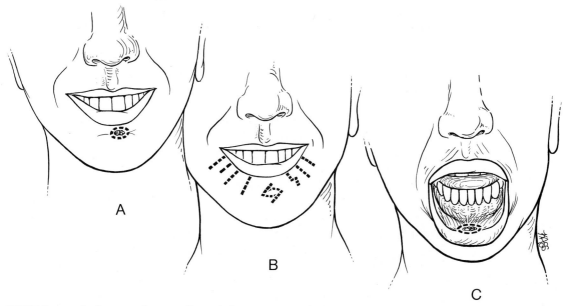

FIGURE 8–3. If a horizontal scar will result from excision of a lesion in the crease between the lower lip and the chin, the surgeon should make a small Z- or W-plasty closure. The area is particularly prone to hypertrophic scar formation because of the horizontal stress that occurs when the patient smiles (*A,B*); otherwise, radial incisions are used. The surgeon can excise lesions of the mucosal surface of the lip (here illustrated as a mucocele excision) transversely or vertically. This is possible because the orbicularis oris muscle influences the dermal scar, and hypertrophic scars are rarely seen on mucosal surfaces (*C*).

eyelid, great care must be taken to observe the position of the eyelid on the limbus after the skin is pinched together.

If distortion of the lid occurs because of inadequate closure of the upper lid, a shift of position of the lower lid on the limbus (scleral show) or a frank ectropion, skin will have to be added. The best method is by adding a full-thickness skin graft either from loose upper lid skin or from the postauricular area.

If the lesion to be excised is deep, a full-thickness excision of the eyelid (skin tarsus conjunctiva) can be accomplished and one third of the eyelid closed primarily (3 to 5 mm). If this is necessary, great care should be taken to align the grey line carefully.

Halving operations or step-like excisions are generally not necessary if proper alignment is made. The sutures near the cornea should be left long and taped to the skin to prevent possible irritation of the cornea. Because of the sensitivity of this area, a 6-0 catgut suture material should be used, as it will approximate the grey line and yet will not require removal.

In closing a full-thickness eyelid excision, the surgeon need not suture the conjunctiva as a separate layer because of the adherence of the underlying tissue. The lid is closed in two layers: A synthetic absorbable suture is used for the tarsal plate, and a monofilament synthetic nonabsorbable suture is used for the skin.

Underlying structures that can be damaged in eyelid surgery are the lacrimal apparatus medially and the levator mechanism superiorly if excisions are too deep. The lacrimal gland, which is at the lateral corner of the upper lid, is usually deep to the orbital rim and is always deep to the septum. Great care must be taken when operating in and around the eyelids to avoid damage to or drying of the cornea. Symptoms of corneal abrasion are a feeling of sand in the eye, coupled with injection of the conjunctiva and epiphora. Lubricants are helpful in preventing this condition in the perioperative period. If a patch is used, it should cause little pressure on the eye. In older patients any stress can precipitate glaucoma. Although it is rare, exceptional pain in the eye, coupled with stony hardness and injected conjunctiva, should be treated as acute onset of glaucoma.

Cheek. The skin of the cheek is thicker and curves over the zygoma (Fig. 8–4). The presence of thick skin means that sutures must be removed early to prevent suture marks. Because of the curve, a W-plasty should be considered for scars that would be longer than 1 to 2 cm. Direct advancement, or, if the skin is too tight, a V-Y flap, works very well in this area. The little flaps of a V-Y scar are quite vascular, and lesions up to 1 or 2 cm can be excised with direct closure, depending on the age of the patient. Again, if the surgeon pinches the skin together, an estimate can be made of the largest amount of tissue that can be excised without

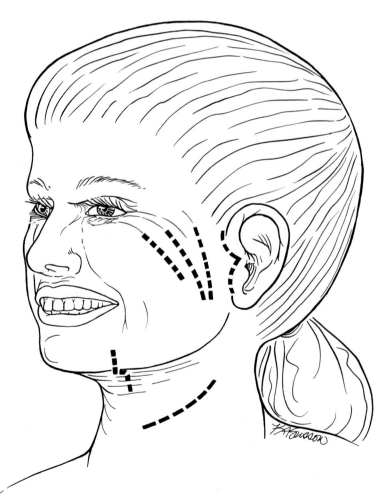

FIGURE 8–4. Direction of facial incisions can be shown by having the patient grimace. Incisions at right angles to the platysma correspond to the transverse lines of the neck. When crossing the border of the mandible, the surgeon should make a step incision. Note that the direction of the muscle changes angles as it goes toward the ear until it is parallel to its long axis. A slight indent at the ear aids in hiding the scar.

distorting the surrounding structures, especially the lower eyelid. As the surgeon moves laterally, the branches of the facial nerve should be considered. Medially, but quite deep, are branches of the maxillary nerve.

Chin. Excisions will vary according to the direction of the muscle pull. Basically, they should be radial in nature. If the scar will go around the corner of the mandible, it should have a zigzag to prevent a bowstring. If the incision is horizontal, a hypertrophic scar commonly forms in the horizontal groove between the lip and chin because of the expansion required in smiling. Radial or zigzag incisions prevent formation of such a scar. The surgeon should be careful of the marginal branch of the seventh cranial nerve when moving laterally from the midline.

Brow. Excisions in the brow should always be beveled to preserve as much brow hair as possible. In making deep excisions, the surgeon needs to avoid the supratrochlear and supraorbital nerves, which emerge from deep in the orbit. Laterally toward the temple and zygoma, branches of the temporal branch of the seventh cranial nerve are superficial. If areas above the brow require an excision of more than 2 or 3 mm, V-Y closure prevents distortion (Fig. 8–5).

The surgeon should be careful to point out pre-existing asymmetry of the brow position (not uncommon, but frequently not noticed by the patient) or to explain that the brow may be distorted later if a larger excision is necessary. Also, one should explain that scars in this area, as in the cheek, take a long time to fade (6 to 18 months in some patients).

Forehead. Horizontal incisions are more easily closed without brow distortion closer to the hairline. V-Y closures are effective in the suprabrow area. Although incisions parallel to the frontalis are preferable, small vertical excisions do not usually cause a problem. All incisions should be parallel to the skin creases. Laterally, the surgeon must watch for the temporal seventh nerve and branches of the temporal artery and medially, for the supraorbital and supratrochlear nerves. If the incision extends into the scalp, the surgeon should bevel the incision to preserve the hair shafts and align the hairline on closure.

Neck. Incisions in the anterior neck should parallel the skin creases, which are at right angles to the direction of pull of the platysma muscle. Posterior neck incisions are also transverse in order to correspond

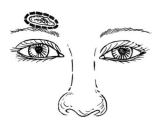
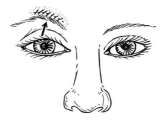
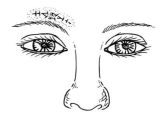

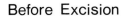

| Before Excision | Incorrect Closure | Correct V-Y Closure |
| A | B | C |

FIGURE 8–5. To prevent distortion of the eyebrow, a subcutaneous V-Y closure (right) is useful after circular excision of a lesion above the brow (left). Distortion may result from direct closure of such a lesion (center).

to the trapezius muscle. There are no structures of concern above the platysma muscle. Deep to the muscle, the seventh and great auricular nerves and the external jugular vein are exposed. The eleventh cranial and the occipital nerves are deep posteriorly.

GROIN

The skin of the groin is thin, and scars should be minor. The incision should be parallel to the crease to reduce the possibility of web formation. The femoral vessels (nerve, artery, vein—lateral to medial) are palpable on the inner aspect but are deep. Superficial branches going to the lower abdomen curve cephalad from below Poupart's ligament. Common lesions include sebaceous cysts, skin tags, and nevi.

AXILLA

The hair-bearing area of the axilla is thin and heals with little scarring. Transverse excisions are preferred in order to reduce the chances of a web formation when the patient abducts the arm. When the arm is abducted, the nerves and vessels of the axilla are in a more superficial position, especially on the brachial surface. In addition, the thoracobrachial nerve (T2) comes from the chest and traverses the axilla to innervate the inner aspect of the arm. Common lesions are sebaceous cysts, skin tags, and nevi. Hidradenitis suppurativa and hyperhydrosis are also conditions in this region treated by more extensive skin excisions.

GENITALIA

Penis. As the skin is quite mobile, large excisions can be made. Many of the rules of skin excision can be violated in this area because of the distensibility of the skin. The preferred incision, however, is transverse rather than longitudinal, because of the expansile nature of the organ. Only small areas of the glands can be excised, because the skin is more rigid. The arteries and nerves are quite superficial on the dorsum, and the urethra is quite superficial on the ventral surface.

Scrotum. The skin is very lax, and large excisions are possible. The skin can be allowed to heal without tight suturing, or even by secondary intention, with excellent results. Infection is rare in this area. The cord and vessels to the testes are easily palpable and can be avoided.

Labia. The tissue of the labia is very much like that of the scrotum. Large excisions can be performed with primary closure, vascularity is excellent, and infection is rare. There are no major structures superficially.

Radial incisions are preferred. Because of rapid healing and the potential for infection, few defects need be sutured. Excisions should be kept very superficial so as not to interfere with the underlying sphincters.

SUMMARY

Incisions should be:
1. Placed at right angles to the direction of the major muscle pull.
2. Allowed to bend.
3. Placed in certain privileged anatomic areas.

PART 4

A Pathologic Approach to Surgery of Common Skin Lesions

chapter 9

BENIGN AND PREMALIGNANT EPIDERMAL SKIN LESIONS

SEBORRHEIC KERATOSES

CLINICAL APPEARANCE

Certainly one of the most common lesions of the skin is the seborrheic keratosis, sometimes referred to as a senile keratosis. This lesion represents an acanthosis or thickening of the malpighian layer of the epidermis.

Clinically, there is an abrupt, well-demarcated border between the seborrheic keratosis and the surrounding skin. This gives the lesion its characteristic stuck-on appearance. Careful inspection reveals that the lesion frequently has a very rough and even warty appearance on the surface. There is a wide variation in color of seborrheic keratoses, ranging from slightly darker than flesh color to a very dark brown or blackish color.

Although any area can be involved with seborrheic keratoses, the palms and soles are always spared, and there is a predilection for involvement of the trunk, face, and scalp. There seems to be some familial tendency to acquiring seborrheic keratoses, and those with this trait tend to develop more as they grow older. Although these lesions can be seen in the third and fourth decade, they are increasingly common after the fifth decade of life.

HISTOPATHOLOGY FOR THE SURGEON

The essential histologic features of the seborrheic keratosis are a thickened stratum corneum (hyperkeratosis), a thickened epidermis (acanthosis), and frequently keratinous horn cysts and pseudohorn cysts. Most lesions have a sharp horizontal demarcation between the lesion and the underlying normal dermis, facilitating removal with a sharp horizontal shearing force. An irritated seborrheic keratosis may show

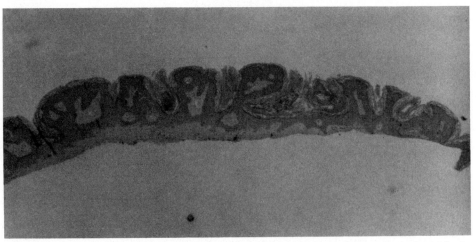

FIGURE 9–1. Histology of seborrheic keratosis showing clear horizontal separation of acanthotic lesion from underlying dermis.

histologic changes similar to a squamous cell carcinoma; however, the presence of epidermal horn cysts and other histologic features and the accurate clinical information supplied by the surgeon can usually rule out true squamous cell carcinoma (Fig. 9–1).

Surgical Treatment

Surgical treatment of seborrheic keratoses is usually done for one of two reasons: (1) cosmetic removal, or (2) differential diagnosis between seborrheic keratosis and any possible malignant lesion, especially of melanocytic origin. A third and less obvious reason for removing such lesions is to clear the skin surface of these easily removed lesions, so that both patient and physician can more accurately observe the skin surface for more suspicious skin growths. In many instances, this proves to be the most important reason for removal of seborrheic keratoses, since patients may frequently have 30 to 40 per cent of the entire skin of the trunk covered with such lesions.

These lesions should not be surgically excised, unless the diagnosis is in question (e.g., melanoma). Removal may be done with a sharp dermal curette. Surgical excision causes unnecessary additional scarring. If the physician does not wish to buy varying sizes of dermal curettes, a No. 3 oval curette will generally suffice for most lesions (e.g., V. Mueller Fox Dermal Curette).

Removal may be done with or without local infiltration of lidocaine, since epidermal curettage is not frequently accompanied by significant pain. I prefer to use 1.0 per cent plain lidocaine locally infiltrated with a 30-gauge needle in small amounts under each keratosis. Curettage is then completely painless (Fig. 9–2).

The edge of the sharp curette is placed firmly against the skin, just distal to one border of the seborrheic keratosis. With the curette angled at approximately 15 to 30 degrees from the horizontal, firm shearing pressure is applied horizontally across the lesion and toward the operator. Such rapid, repetitive movements will easily remove the seborrheic keratosis at the epidermal junction. The operator will clearly see a *smooth superficial dermis* (Figs. 9–3 and 9–4).

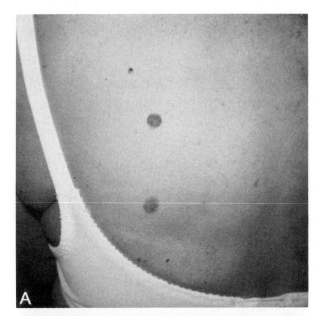

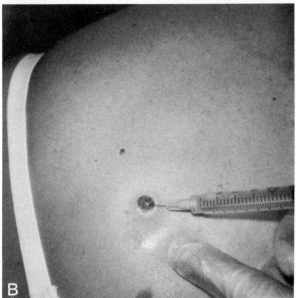

FIGURE 9–2. *A*, Typical seborrheic keratoses on back. *B*, Superficial infiltration of keratosis with a 30-gauge needle, causing a wheal and virtually immediate anesthesia.

This immediately provides the operator with a firm diagnosis of a strictly epidermal lesion, as compared to melanoma or other dermal tumors, which would have deeper connections in the skin. If there is any question of the diagnosis before or just after starting curettage, excision may be performed.

Even strictly epidermal lesions such as an epidermal nevus will not be removed with such a clean base after curettage. This is because of interdigitating dermal papillae projecting upward between epidermal proliferations. A seborrheic keratosis usually has a distinct sharp horizontal border with the underlying dermis. In most instances, the operator will be able to rapidly diagnose the lesion as a seborrheic keratosis and with experience even avoid submitting such a specimen for histopatho-

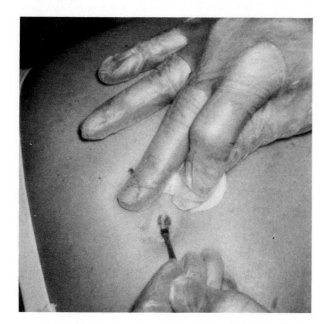

FIGURE 9–3. Curette easily removes part of seborrheic keratosis, showing smooth white dermis underneath.

logic examination; however, medical-legal circumstances may dictate otherwise. If the diagnosis is certain and there is some resistance to curette removal, light electrodesiccation before removal facilitates separation of the seborrheic keratosis from underlying dermis (Fig. 9–4C to E).

After removal with the curette, the operator will notice several punctate, bleeding superficial dermal blood vessels. Although electrocautery may suffice for hemostasis in such instances, a skin burn, albeit infrequent, is a classic injury for induction of hypertrophic scar in patients so predisposed. For this reason, I use a 35 per cent solution of aluminum chloride in 50 per cent isopropyl alcohol as a quick-acting styptic (Fig. 9–5). This eliminates the possible scarring secondary to electrocautery and avoids the pigmentation seen with other styptics, such as Monsel's solution and silver nitrate. The resulting superficially abraded skin may be left open to heal, with gentle superficial cleansing with hydrogen peroxide or 70 per cent isopropyl alcohol twice daily. The result will usually be complete healing with little or no visible scar.

Other methods using either heat or cold (electrosurgery and cryosurgery) may not give such consistently good cosmetic results. Such methods rely upon using sufficient heat or cold to cause epidermal separation, but not enough to cause deeper dermal destruction and scarring. Since individuals vary greatly in their response to heat or cold and since different areas of the body have differing sensitivities, the accuracy of removal by these methods is less controlled with respect to the depth of injury and possible scar formation. I find much better control and less visible reaction with light electrodesiccation than with cryosurgery. A very slightly charred surface after light electrodesiccation seems to heal more predictably than after cryosurgery, in which small, large, or no blisters may result from the same application in different patients. It is obvious by the results obtained with curettage (Fig. 9–6) that excisions should be avoided for seborrheic keratoses.

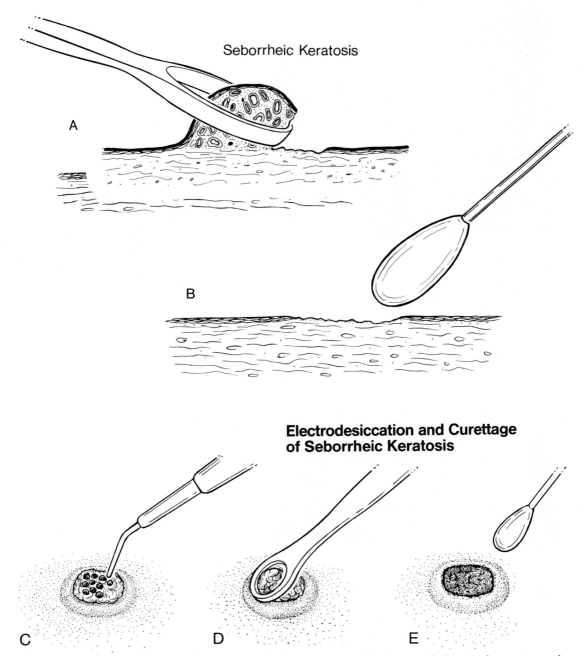

Seborrheic Keratosis

Electrodesiccation and Curettage of Seborrheic Keratosis

FIGURE 9–4. *A* and *B*, Curette easily removes seborrheic keratosis with horizontal shearing force. A smooth white glistening superficial dermis is seen on the surface now. *C* to *E*, Light electrodesiccation before curettage of seborrheic keratosis facilitates epidermal-dermal separation for smooth, clean removal with curette.

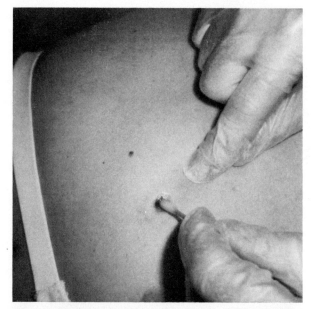

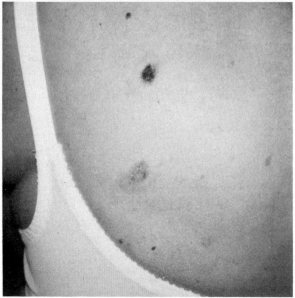

FIGURE 9–5. *A,* Thirty-five per cent aluminum chloride styptic is applied to the bleeding base after curettage of the seborrheic keratosis. *B,* Complete hemostasis achieved with styptic after curettage of two seborrheic keratoses.

WARTS (VERRUCA VULGARIS)

CLINICAL APPEARANCE

Warts represent an epidermal proliferation as a result of skin being infected with the human papilloma virus. They are frequently separated into different clinical groups, either by morphologic appearance or by location on the skin surface.

Filiform warts have many fine villous-type projections, usually grouped tightly together in one lesion. Such warts are more common on the face and extremities. Flat warts seem to be more common on the hands and the face and are usually skin colored or slightly brownish. Flat warts frequently are present in great numbers. Plantar warts are

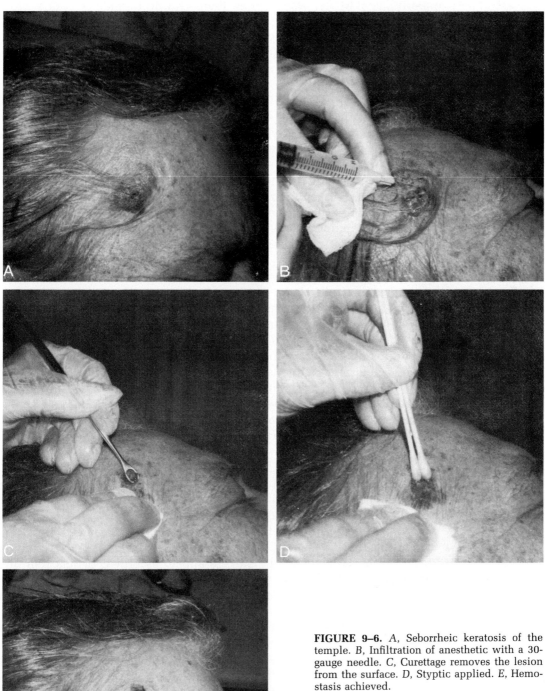

FIGURE 9–6. *A,* Seborrheic keratosis of the temple. *B,* Infiltration of anesthetic with a 30-gauge needle. *C,* Curettage removes the lesion from the surface. *D,* Styptic applied. *E,* Hemostasis achieved.

usually filiform warts that have been flattened and pressed into the underlying skin by walking on them. Multiple plantar warts close together, termed mosaic warts, are very difficult to treat. Condylomata acuminata are warts usually found in the genital or perianal area. Such warts are also frequently filiform and characterized by a moist surface. The most common (but not exclusive) means of transferring condylomata is by sexual contact.

Most areas of the skin surface may be involved with the wart virus, but the hands, face, genital-anal area, and plantar surface of the feet are the most commonly involved. The trunk and proximal extremities are much less frequently involved.

Although warts are seen at all ages, they occur most frequently in childhood and early adult life. There does seem to be some tendency to transfer warts between family members.

A particularly important type of warty growth called epidermodysplasia verruciformis seems to be inherited and has the potential of changing into squamous cell carcinoma. For the most part, the average wart does not have such malignant potential. Giant condyloma of Buschke, usually located on the penis, is also a lesion with potential to form squamous cell carcinoma.

It has been said that many warts will involute on their own without treatment in approximately two years. There is considerable variation in such resolution (which may never occur), and, therefore, most dermatologists favor removing existing warts to prevent both further cosmetic deformity with the growth of additional warts on the patient and transfer of warts to other family members. A large condyloma, persistent genital warts, persistent flat warts with a familial history, and warts of prolonged duration despite treatment should probably be biopsied to rule out squamous cell carcinoma.

HISTOPATHOLOGY FOR THE SURGEON

Hyperkeratosis, acanthosis, and papillomatosis are usually seen. Vacuolated virus-infiltrated epidermal cells in areas of parakeratosis are seen in the upper epidermis and stratum corneum. Well-vascularized dermal papillae protrude upward into areas of thickened epidermis, accounting for the usually profuse bleeding during surgical removal. Thrombosed vessels near the surface appear as brown or blackish dots clinically. A variable degree of inflammation, usually of predominantly monocytic cell line, may be seen in the dermis (especially in resolving flat warts).

Close pathologic examination should be done for persistent genital warts (especially a large condyloma or warts present for two years or more) for bowenoid changes. It is a good idea to get a pathologic specimen that includes the dermis (to identify any squamous cell invasion). If a biopsy is to be done, it should be prior to or significantly after any application of podophyllum to the lesion, since podophyllum can induce bowenoid changes.

Atypical verrucous lesions and persistent lesions not responding to treatment (especially on the plantar surface of the foot) should be biopsied to rule out verrucous carcinoma. Extensive flat warts not responding to treatment (especially with a familial occurrence) should make one suspicious of epidermodysplasia verruciformis, which may develop into carcinoma in some warts. Atypical changes should be promptly biopsied. Select laboratories will also type the wart virus to confirm the suspicion of epidermodysplasia verruciformis.

SURGICAL TREATMENT

Dozens of effective treatments for warts exist today. Although the lesion is limited to the epidermis, there are dermal papillae interdigitating between epidermal ridges, making it difficult to achieve a clean separation between epidermis and dermis (Fig. 9–7). Therapy is directed at local destruction of the epidermis containing the wart virus, allowing re-epithelialization with uninfected epidermis.

The most common methods used are acids, cryotherapy, and electrodesiccation and curettage. Trichloroacetic acid in strengths from 35 to 80 per cent may be applied at weekly intervals at the office and covered with an occlusive tape such as Blenderm. This may be used in conjunction with other acids applied daily at home, such as a compound of 16 per cent lactic acid and 16 per cent salicylic acid in flexible collodion. Occlusion with Blenderm or adhesive tape over the acid usually facilitates penetration. The warts should be pared once or twice weekly with such acid treatments. The depth of penetration should be followed closely so that acid does not penetrate beyond wart-infected epidermis.

For plantar warts, 40 per cent salicylic acid impregnated in an adhesive plaster is frequently used. Such a plaster may be applied to the

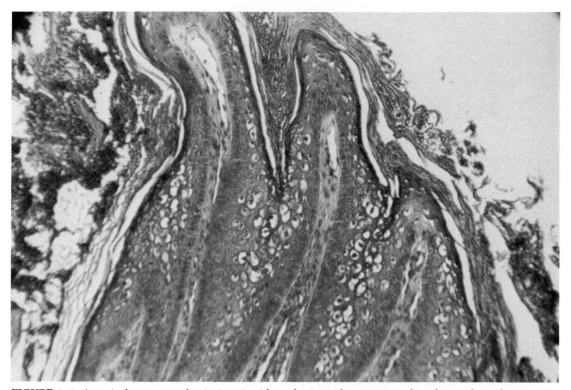

FIGURE 9–7. A typical verruca vulgaris (wart) with no horizontal separation of epidermis from dermis as in seborrheic keratoses.

wart's surface and covered with adhesive tape. It may be removed every two or three days with subsequent paring or curettage of the wart. Care again should be taken not to allow penetration deeper than the wart itself (Fig. 9–8).

Moist warts in the genital area (condylomata acuminata) may be treated with 20 or 25 per cent podophyllum in a tincture of benzoin. Such treatment may be carried out on a weekly basis in the office. Podophyllum should be applied only to the wart surface and not to a large area at one time because of possible systemic absorption and side effects (Fig. 9–9). Meticulous care should be used when applying such medication, and petrolatum or an appropriate protective ointment or paste may be placed on surrounding normal skin. Podophyllum may be left on for one to twelve hours and washed off in a sitz bath. There have been reports of bowenoid changes in warts treated with podophyllum, so that on subsequent histologic examination the lesion may be difficult to differentiate from de novo bowenoid papules. Podophyllum is a strong DNA poison and should be used only by the physician with close follow-up.

Cryotherapy or freezing of warts with either liquid nitrogen or carbon dioxide is a very common and acceptable form of treatment (Fig.

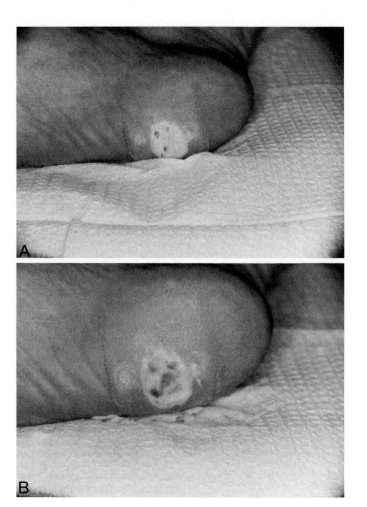

FIGURE 9–8. Forty per cent salicylic acid plaster applied to plantar wart. Tape will be placed over this. *A,* Moist white tissue created by two days of 40 per cent salicylic acid plaster. *B,* Defect remaining after removal of wart tissue.

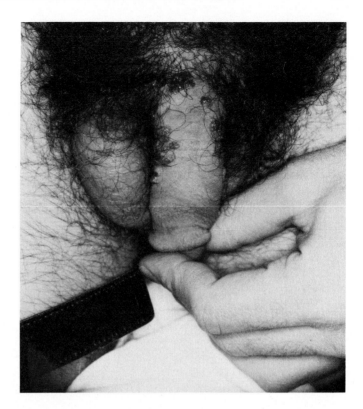

FIGURE 9–9. Application of 25 per cent podophyllum in tincture of benzoin to condyloma.

9–10). The one major drawback of any cryotherapy is the great variability of cold sensitivity of different patients and different surface locations. Some patients may form large bullae within only a second or two of application with liquid nitrogen or carbon dioxide ice. This may limit the predictability of such treatment. It has been said by some that cryotherapy is essentially free of scarring. This is completely untrue, and the potential for scarring with cryotherapy is as clear and real as its potential for causing dermal injury. The purpose of cryotherapy is to cause a small blister. It is hoped that the wart will fall off when the top of the blister does. Under the proper circumstances this leaves excellent cosmetic results. It is the treatment of choice for many dermatologists.

Electrodesiccation with curettage is also an acceptable method of treatment for warts, but only if secondary scarring from the procedure is acceptable. Since a developing scar may become painful, it is usually inadvisable to use this method first for large warts on the plantar surface on the feet. The scar created in this location may be a permanent disability. These are only relative contraindications weighed against the rapid and thorough removal achievable with electrodesiccation (Fig. 9–10B to G).

Local infiltration of plain lidocaine 1 per cent is followed by moderate electrodesiccation of the warts. The desiccated wart is removed with a sharp curette or Gradle scissors. Brisk bleeding is frequently encountered with this removal and may be decreased or stopped with application of 35 per cent aluminum chloride solution. This provides better visualization of tissue before further destruction by electrodesiccation. If the wart clearly remains, additional light electrodesiccation

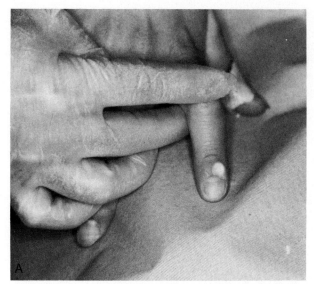

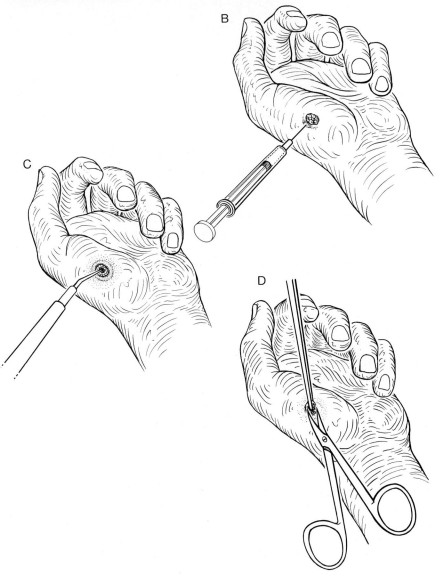

FIGURE 9–10. *A,* Freezing a wart with liquid nitrogen spray. *B* to *G,* Steps in the electrodesiccation of a wart.

Illustration continued on opposite page

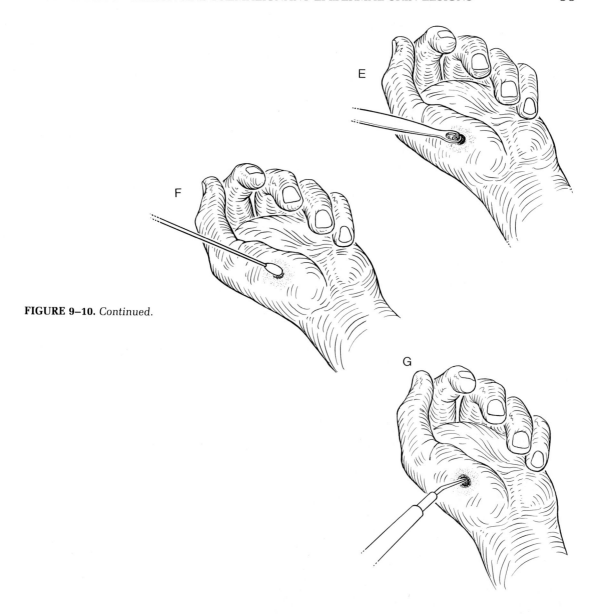

FIGURE 9–10. *Continued.*

may be used, care being taken not to electrodesiccate deep dermal tissue, which may cause scarring.

A great advantage of this method is the use of sharp fine scissors (Gradle, etc.) and the curette to determine exactly how deeply and widely wart tissue extends. A good operator easily learns to recognize healthy smooth dermis and stops dissection and desiccation at that level. Electrodesiccation is used only to facilitate removal of the bulk of the wart and to lightly cauterize to prevent recurrence after removal. Hemostasis is achieved mainly with aluminum chloride solution. Chemical and freezing methods lack this exact determination of depth and width and, therefore, are more prone to undertreat or overtreat depending upon the extent of treatment and patient response.

Warts may recur with any of the above treatments, but persistent failure with one modality may be followed by quick resolution with one of the others. Most methods have about a 70 per cent success rate.

ACTINIC KERATOSIS

CLINICAL DESCRIPTION

The synonym for this lesion is solar keratosis, as its cause is excessive exposure to the sun. These lesions are adherent, variably keratotic, epidermal growths. They are usually a whitish or flesh color with or without inflammation but may also be a tan or yellowish color. Perhaps the most common presentation is an erythematous base with a clear to whitish thickened keratin that can be felt as a rough area when passing the fingertips across the skin surface (Fig. 9–11).

The dorsal aspect of the hands, the arms, the face, and the scalp (in balding patients) are most frequently involved. These lesions may begin as early as the third decade but are more frequently seen in the sixth decade or later, with increasing numbers as the patient ages. There is a definite tendency for those with light skin and blue eyes (especially those of Celtic ancestry) to acquire such lesions. There is also a probable familial predisposition, but the extent of sun exposure over the patient's life will make expression of this greatly variable.

These lesions are premalignant and will, over a long period of time, have the potential for developing into a squamous cell carcinoma. It is for this reason that treatment is uniformly recommended. Squamous cell carcinoma arising in these lesions rarely is aggressive or metastatic when detected early. This is in sharp distinction to squamous cell

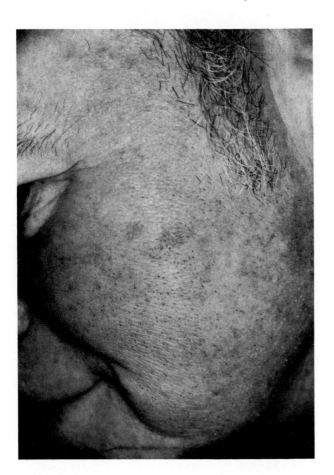

FIGURE 9–11. Slight roughness representing hyperkeratosis on an erythematous base, a typical actinic keratosis.

carcinoma arising de novo, from chronic draining ulcers or sinuses, from mucous membranes, from Bowen's disease, or from burn scars. The majority of actinic keratoses will not degenerate into squamous cell carcinoma, and the ones that will usually do so only after several years.

HISTOPATHOLOGY FOR THE SURGEON

Variable thickening of the stratum corneum (hyperkeratosis) may be seen. The atrophic variety may have only a thin scale clinically, while a hypertrophic variety may form a cutaneous horn. A disorderly appearance to the cells of the stratum malpighii is characteristic, with accompanying anaplastic nuclei and pleomorphism. Dyskeratosis may also be seen and may result in spaces or lacunae between cells. Proliferation of the basal layer in bud-shaped projections into the dermis is also frequently seen.

The above changes are usually more scattered and less pronounced than with squamous cell carcinoma in situ (Bowen's disease). Because of the sun-induced nature of these lesions a variable amount of elastotic solar degeneration of collagen is usually present. Collagen may appear bluish on routine hematoxylin and eosin sections.

Perhaps the most important reason for the surgeon to recognize the essential pathologic features of the actinic keratosis is identification of such changes in epidermis adjacent to or in a developing squamous cell carcinoma. Corroborating clinical information may identify a squamous cell carcinoma arising from an actinic keratosis and thus place it in a less aggressive malignant category with a low incidence of metastasis, allowing less aggressive or deforming surgical treatment.

SURGICAL TREATMENT

Curettage and electrodesiccation, cryosurgery, and topical 5-fluorouracil are all acceptable methods of removing actinic keratoses. Curettage and electrodesiccation are perhaps the most definitive of the above methods.

The heat of electrodesiccation causes a separation of the epidermis from the dermis. The curette will accurately determine complete removal of the actinic keratosis, and subsequent light electrodesiccation will provide sufficient destruction of dysplastic epidermis and adjacent superficial dermis. Curettage also may enable the operator to determine whether there is any growth, such as a squamous cell carcinoma, penetrating beyond the superficial actinic keratosis. This may be manifested by a soft gelatinous type of material underneath the superficial keratosis, as compared to normal firm dermis.

Such clinical assessment of underlying tissue is not available with cryosurgery or topical chemotherapy. Although cryosurgery is quick and easy, it again has the problem of determining just how much is necessary for removal of the lesion, avoiding too much or too little freezing in that particular individual for that particular skin surface area. It is, however, my treatment of choice for superficial actinic keratoses.

The use of topical 5-fluorouracil creams and solutions over large areas of actinic damaged skin has been advocated by many. It seems that this method will "light up" clinically undetectable actinic keratoses during treatment (Fig. 9–12). The lesions themselves and also surrounding normal skin may become quite inflamed during twice-a-day treatment

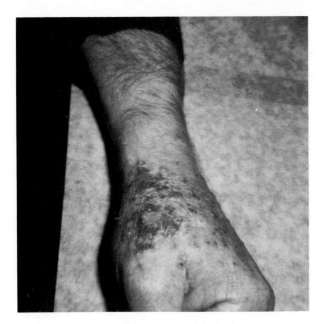

FIGURE 9–12. Two per cent topical 5-fluorouracil has caused undetected premalignant areas to "light-up" in this patient. Only a few keratoses were clinically visible before treatment.

with such topical creams and solutions in 2 per cent and 5 per cent concentrations. Treatment is usually necessary for three weeks or longer, sometimes contributing to significant cosmetic problems for the individual patient. Topical steroid creams and ointments may also be used during treatment to decrease inflammation. This does not seem to decrease the effectiveness of the 5-fluorouracil.

When extensive actinic degeneration and actinic keratoses preceding squamous cell carcinoma are present on the face, an excellent method of treatment is dermabrasion. Superficial dermabrasion will effectively remove existing actinic keratoses and also surrounding sun-damaged epidermis. Since this treatment does not necessitate deep dermabrasion, crusts may be off after only one week's time with smooth, pink skin underlying this. Cosmetic results of dermabrasion for sun-damaged skin are distinctly superior and perhaps are the most esthetically satisfactory results obtained with dermabrasion for any reason.

Except in the case of developing squamous cell carcinoma, excision is usually unnecessary for actinic keratosis where removal of underlying dermis or fat is not indicated. Also, most patients will develop multiple lesions, so scarring from surgery should be kept to a minimum.

LENTIGO SENILIS

CLINICAL DESCRIPTION

Lentigo senilis or senile lentigines are the commonly mentioned "age spots" usually occurring on sun-exposed skin surfaces. Such lesions are rather permanent and do not have as much fluctuation in coloration with sun exposure, as freckles (ephelides) do. These lesions occur with increasing frequency with age (Fig. 9–13).

They represent only a mild thickening of the epidermis in some layers and increased pigment formation of the epidermis in that particular area. These lesions are entirely epidermal and should not be excised. If

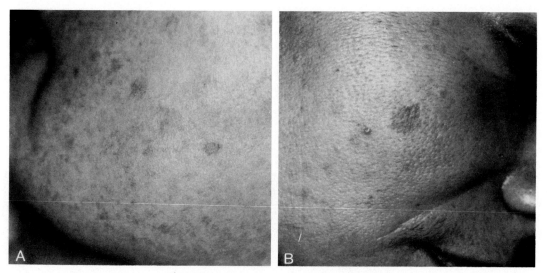

FIGURE 9–13. Examples of lentigo senilis.

there is question as to the diagnosis of such a lesion, a small biopsy may be done.

HISTOPATHOLOGY FOR THE SURGEON

The epidermis shows elongation of rete ridges, usually with bud-shaped proliferations. An increased number of melanocytes and pigment formation account for the darker color of these lesions.

SURGICAL TREATMENT

Since surgical removal is cosmetic only, whatever method of removal is chosen should be done slowly and carefully in a restricted area first. If approached slowly, cryosurgery is perhaps the best method available. Either solid carbon dioxide sticks or liquid nitrogen spray should be used very cautiously to begin and should be restricted to the area of increased hyperpigmentation (Fig. 9–14A and B). All attempts should be made to avoid blistering. One must also be careful not to cause exaggerated hypopigmentation of the lentiginous area, as compared to the surrounding normally pigmented skin. Carbon dioxide is not as cold ($-79°C$) as liquid nitrogen ($-196°C$), allowing the operator to vary the time and pressure of application more for greater control with carbon dioxide. Prolonged application will cause hypopigmentation, while too brief an application may result in greater pigmentation. Very superficial curettage with a sharp curette may also be performed but should not be followed by electrodesiccation. Aluminum chloride as a styptic following such curettage is acceptable for hemostasis.

Use of varying percentages of trichloroacetic acid is also an acceptable method for such lesions. Again, one should begin with low percentages of trichloroacetic acid (e.g., 25 per cent) applied for short periods of time and proceed slowly.

Bleaching creams, such as hydroquinones, applied by the patient daily can achieve good results in some patients. A compounded cream of equal parts hydroquinone cream 4 per cent, vitamin A acid cream (Retin-A) 0.1 per cent, and hydrocortisone cream 2.5 per cent may be

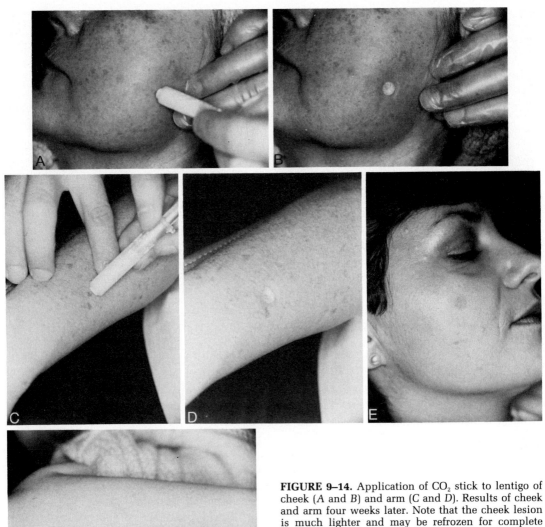

FIGURE 9–14. Application of CO_2 stick to lentigo of cheek (*A* and *B*) and arm (*C* and *D*). Results of cheek and arm four weeks later. Note that the cheek lesion is much lighter and may be refrozen for complete removal, but cosmetics now cover the lesion easily. *E* and *F*, Result four weeks later in another patient.

applied b.i.d. to start. If irritation or extensive depigmentation does not result, the hydrocortisone may be eliminated. This therapy takes several weeks. Stronger hydroquinone creams may be helpful in the future. Very potent strengths (e.g., 20 per cent) will permanently depigment skin and should not be used.

EPIDERMAL NEVI

CLINICAL DESCRIPTION

Epidermal nevi are the result of a developmental abnormality and are usually present at birth or emerge in early childhood. Recent evidence seems to indicate that other internal abnormalities (especially of the

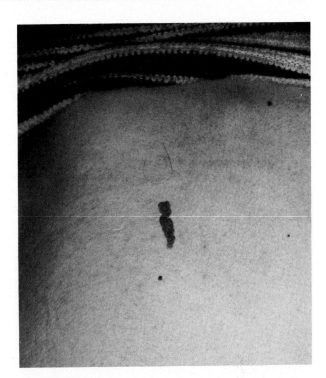

FIGURE 9–15. Epidermal nevus on the back.

central nervous system) may be associated in some circumstances with epidermal nevi.

They are usually verrucous and light to dark brown in color (Fig. 9–15). Although they are also entirely epidermal, they do not have the stuck-on appearance of seborrheic keratoses. Although they themselves are usually benign, internal developmental abnormalities may cause functional defects.

HISTOPATHOLOGY FOR THE SURGEON

The essential features are variable hyperkeratosis, acanthosis, and papillomatosis. The papillomatosis (dermal papillae projecting upward between thickened epidermal rete ridges) clearly distinguishes this lesion from a seborrheic keratosis, which has a clear horizontal thickening of the epidermis. Such papillomatosis prevents easy removal of the epidermal lesion with the horizontal shearing force of the curette.

SURGICAL TREATMENT

Because there is not a clear-cut horizontal border between the epidermis and dermis with epidermal nevi, they are not as easily removed with superficial shaving methods, curettage, or dermabrasion. The most satisfactory method of removal for epidermal nevi is excisional surgery. These lesions are not generally malignant in character, and the best possible cosmetic results should be the goal in treatment.

ARSENICAL KERATOSES

Arsenical keratoses are keratotic growths occurring on the palms and the soles of people who have been exposed to arsenic as long as 20 years or more previously. Since these lesions are premalignant, they should be removed or closely followed. Superficial destructive methods or excision (when possible) should be done. Histopathologic examination of specimens should be done to rule out invasive squamous cell carcinoma. (See Chapter 12 for further discussion of malignant skin lesions.)

CUTANEOUS HORNS

CLINICAL DESCRIPTION

Many different underlying pathologic processes are represented clinically as a cutaneous horn. This usually presents as a very thick, vertical accumulation of keratinous material projecting from the skin

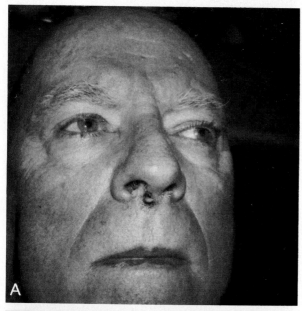

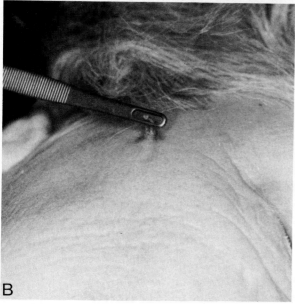

FIGURE 9–16. *A*, Cutaneous horn under right nostril. *B*, Cutaneous horn on right cheek.

surface in a similar manner to an animal's horn (Fig. 9–16). Such lesions are more frequently found on sun-exposed skin areas. They tend to occur more in the fourth decade or later, but they may occur at any age.

HISTOPATHOLOGY FOR THE SURGEON

The cutaneous horn is simply an accumulation of keratinous material overlying any one of a number of different histopathologic entities. Cutaneous horns may cover such pathologic entities as seborrheic keratoses, arsenical keratoses, actinic keratoses, squamous cell carcinoma, and warts.

SURGICAL TREATMENT

Because many different benign and malignant tumors may produce cutaneous horns, complete excision with examination of the total histopathologic specimen is necessary. Superficial destructive methods that do not give an adequate histopathologic specimen may miss invasive malignancy and should be avoided.

If the cutaneous horn is over a finger or other area where conservation of tissue is of primary importance, an initial superficial shave biopsy may be done with care, extending somewhat into the superficial dermis to detect invasion into deeper layers of the skin. If a totally benign lesion limited to the epidermis, such as a seborrheic keratosis, is found on microscopic examination of such a biopsy, no further specimen is necessary. If there is any evidence of deeper invasion, the surgeon must return for a deeper and more thorough biopsy.

chapter 10

BENIGN DERMAL SKIN LESIONS

NEVOCELLULAR NEVI

CLINICAL DESCRIPTION

The most common form of nevi, which the laity refer to as moles, can be conveniently grouped into three different types:

1. Intradermal nevi—these lesions are usually elevated above the surrounding skin surface and do not have a macular (flat) pigmented component (Fig. 10–1).
2. Junctional nevi—these nevi have pigmented nevus cells within the epidermis, giving a clinical appearance of a macular (flat) pigmented lesion (Fig. 10–2).
3. Compound nevi—these nevi have the clinical appearance of both intradermal and junctional nevi, frequently with both an elevated component and a macular pigmented component often seen extending beyond the border of the intradermal component (Fig. 10–3).

With the exception of congenital nevi, most nevi begin to occur in childhood and progress through early adulthood. After the third decade, the frequency of occurrence of new nevi decreases.

There does seem to be a definite familial tendency toward developing multiple nevi. A recently recognized syndrome (dysplastic nevus syndrome) has been identified in which multiple nevi with irregular colors and shapes, located mostly on the trunk, have a higher incidence of development of malignant melanoma. This finding has lead many dermatologists to recommend removal of suspicious nevi, perhaps with greater frequency in these families.

HISTOPATHOLOGY FOR THE SURGEON

Nevocellular nevi are mostly an aggregation of melanocytic nevus cells in the epidermis and the dermis. Close examination of any suspicious lesion should be done with serial sections. The seriousness of a

109

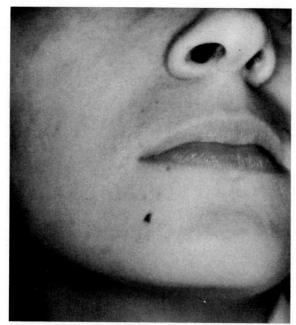

A

FIGURE 10–1. Intradermal nevus.

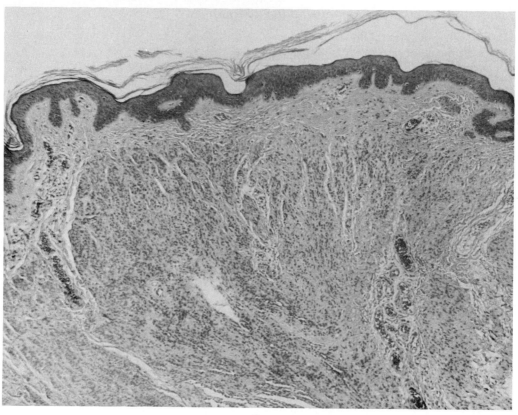

B

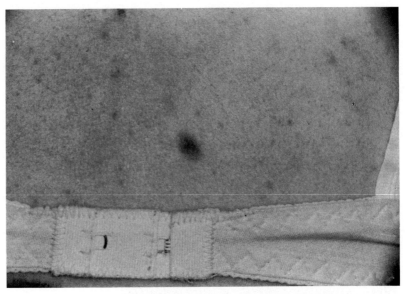

FIGURE 10–2. Junctional nevus.

melanocytic malignancy should prompt histologic examination of all nevi surgically removed.

Tumor thickness is extremely important as a prognostic indicator in melanoma. It will also affect the type and extent of treatment of the melanoma. When melanoma is considered, removal to at least the subcutaneous fat or superficial fascia is preferable. Any specimen not showing complete tumor thickness may destroy this valuable histologic parameter. Shave type biopsies, therefore, should be avoided when melanoma is suspected.

SURGICAL TREATMENT

Nevocellular nevi are usually removed for one of the following three reasons: (1) cosmetic improvement; (2) to rule out or prevent the development of malignant melanoma in a suspicious or congenital lesion; (3) to prevent continual irritation and inflammation in a trauma- or friction-prone area.

Two acceptable methods for removing nevi for cosmetic reasons are frequently used. If a nevus is pedunculated or markedly elevated from the surrounding skin, an attempt may be made to shave the lesion flush or just below the surface. Such a procedure frequently removes all or most of the existing pigment and also removes all or most of the aesthetically unacceptable portion of the nevus (Fig. 10–4). This method may leave a portion of the nevus within the dermis and, therefore, may be an incomplete removal (Fig. 10–5A to C). If there is a suspicion of malignancy, this method should not be used.

The remaining nevus within the skin may also repigment heavily and irregularly, giving an unacceptable cosmetic result (Fig. 10–6). If this happens, excision of the remaining nevus may then be done. With this shaving procedure, it is important to let the patient know that the nevus is not being completely removed. Patients may subsequently have the shaved nevus looked at by another physician with submission of a

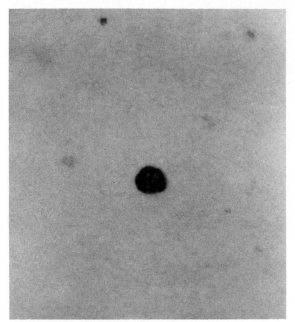

A

FIGURE 10–3. Compound nevus.

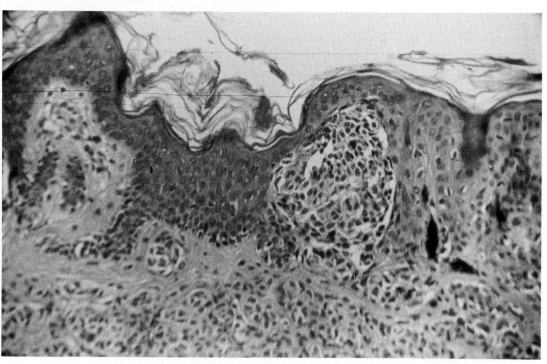

B

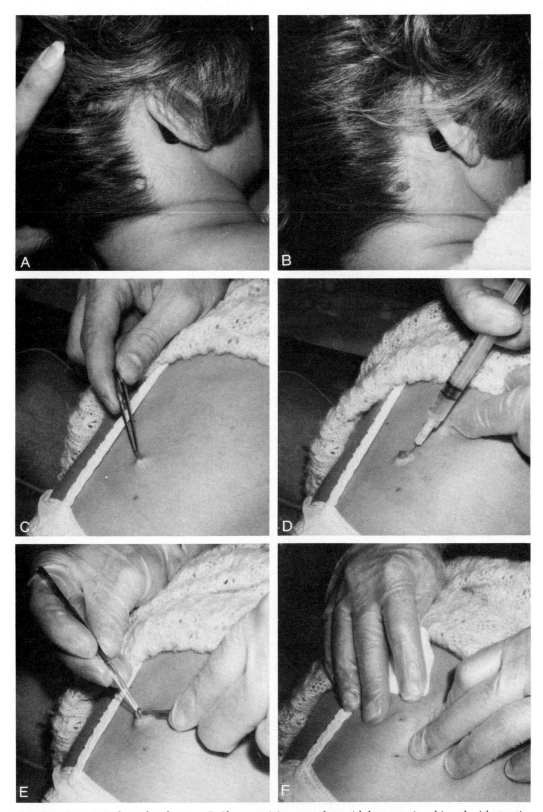

FIGURE 10–4. *A*, Pedunculated nevus. *B*, Shave excision complete with hemostasis achieved with styptic. *C*, Forceps holding pedunculated nevus. *D*, Infiltration of anesthetic around pedunculated nevus. *E*, Scalpel shaves nevus parallel to surface. *F*, Hemostasis achieved with styptic.

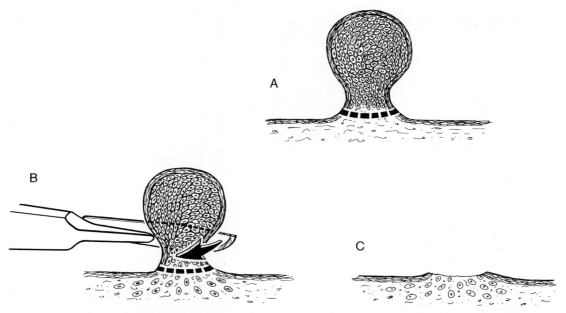

FIGURE 10–5. *A,* Pedunculated intradermal nevus with all nevus cells above surrounding skin surface. *B,* Pedunculated nevus with some nevus cells below surface of surrounding skin. *C,* Incomplete removal of all nevus cells by shave removal of lesion in *B.*

histopathologic specimen that is altered. Awareness by the patient of the technique used may eliminate possible questions of atypical clinical and histopathologic features.

Despite the disadvantages of the shave method, two advantages do exist. If the nevus is of significantly large diameter, a shave may leave a more acceptable scar if the surface is left flat and relatively unpigmented. If an unacceptable result is obtained, the lesion may always be excised, whereas, if it is excised first, an unacceptable result in that circumstance cannot be shaved. The other advantage to such a method is that in areas such as the sternum and deltoid area, where scarring from excisional

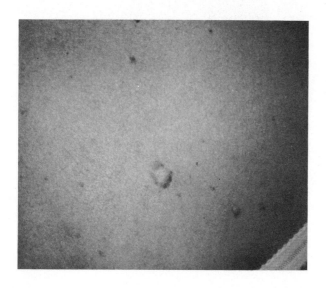

FIGURE 10–6. Irregular pigment occurring around a nevus that was shaved by another physician years before.

surgery is less than optimum, the shave procedure may leave superior cosmetic results.

When performing any shave excision of a nevus, the physician should take extreme care to shave the nevus flat or just below the surrounding skin. The operator must be very careful to avoid shaving either too deep or too superficially. Occasionally, if a rough border exists after shaving, a sharp curette may be used to even out the borders. Shave excision can usually be followed with a simple aluminum chloride styptic, although light electrodesiccation may also be used.

Any nevus with a recent change in size, sensation, color, or other physical characteristic, should be completely excised so that histopathologic exam in toto can be completed. Any recently traumatized, bleeding, or ulcerated lesions should obviously be excised. Excision is a perfectly acceptable, and in many cases superior, surgical technique for removal of nevocellular nevi (Fig. 10–7). As mentioned above, it may also follow unsatisfactory cosmetic results obtained with a shave excision.

Unless the lesion is extremely suspicious for melanoma, the margin of the excision should be the visible clinical border of the nevus. If malignant melanoma is strongly suspected, the surgeon may wish to take several extra millimeters even at the initial excisional biopsy. Although no definite evidence exists for cancer spread with incisional biopsies extending through malignant melanoma, most surgeons would agree that an excisional biopsy extending beyond the clinical border in width and depth is preferable. If malignant melanoma is suspected, the excision should be taken to the depth of subcutaneous tissue or superficial fascia. When possible, excision lines should be in the direction of lymphatic flow, as this may be the direction of future surgical excision in some circumstances.

It is well-known that congenital giant nevi have an increased incidence of malignant degeneration. A controversy exists, however, over whether smaller congenital nevi have such increased malignant potential. Extensive data are not available on this subject to date but will, it is hoped, be accumulated prospectively. It has been suggested by some that only congenital nevi greater than 1.5 cm in diameter should be excised. Sufficient factual data not being available, it seems wise to prophylactically excise all congenital nevi, since smaller lesions are frequently excised with excellent cosmetic result. This view has gained considerable support in recent years. Only one out of 100 to 200 newborn infants has congenital nevi. A recent study by Rhodes et al. (1982) does lend significant support to the idea that even small congenital nevi have a higher incidence of malignant melanoma formation. Data such as these have recently led to a recommendation by some to excise all congenital nevocellular nevi (Arons and Hurwitz, 1983).

I recently saw melanomas develop in small congenital nevi in two males (ages 21 and 52) in the same two-week period. I could not help thinking of what benefit prophylactic excision might have offered. The melanoma in the 52-year-old man was Stage IV and almost 1 cm thick, with a very poor prognosis.

As mentioned above, the dysplastic nevus syndrome seems to be a more common entity in families with an inherited pattern of multiple nevi (Fig. 10–8). These nevi are frequently present in large numbers with

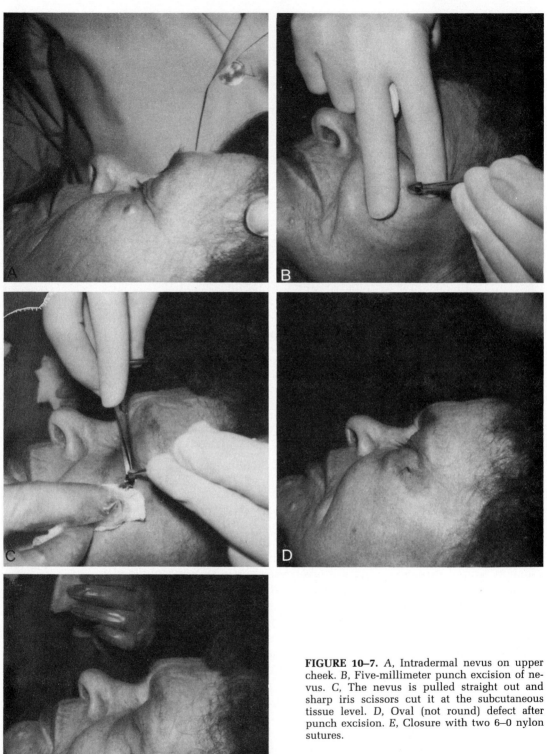

FIGURE 10–7. *A*, Intradermal nevus on upper cheek. *B*, Five-millimeter punch excision of nevus. *C*, The nevus is pulled straight out and sharp iris scissors cut it at the subcutaneous tissue level. *D*, Oval (not round) defect after punch excision. *E*, Closure with two 6–0 nylon sutures.

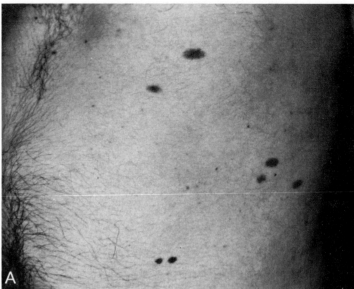

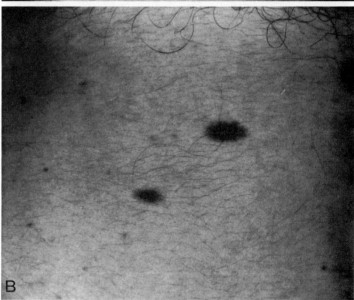

FIGURE 10–8. Patient with dysplastic nevi. Irregular border seen in *B*.

varying sizes, shapes, and colors. Because of an increased incidence of melanoma in these families, the surgeon must have an increased awareness of the possibility of malignant degeneration in any patient with an inherited pattern of such nevi. Early removal with complete excision at the sign of any suspicious change should be done. Close follow-up with photographs has been recommended by some; however, I prefer to excise any nevus suspicious enough to warrant frequent photographs. Although the cost and time of such surgery can easily be discussed at medical meetings, it is much more difficult to justify such concerns when advising an individual patient face to face. I would not photograph my own suspicious nevi but have them excised in toto. Nevus cells under the microscope will not turn malignant!

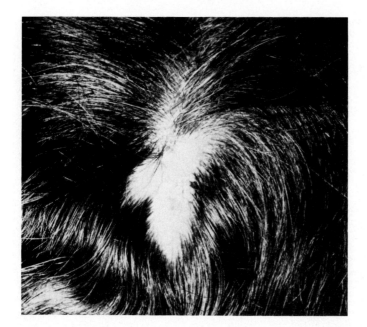

FIGURE 10–9. Sebaceous nevus. (Photo courtesy of Nancy B. Esterly, M.D.)

SEBACEOUS NEVUS OF JADASSOHN

CLINICAL DESCRIPTION

The sebaceous nevus usually presents at birth or early in childhood with a flesh-colored to yellowish or yellowish-brown pebbly appearance, frequently on the scalp. It may often clinically resemble an epidermal nevus (Fig. 10–9). Although originally composed of benign components, a sebaceous nevus does have pluripotential cells that may develop into other benign tumors such as a syringocystadenoma papilliferum or malignant lesions such as basal cell carcinoma. A higher degree of malignant degeneration seems to occur around puberty, and, therefore, most lesions should be removed before that time.

HISTOPATHOLOGY FOR THE SURGEON

In early life there may be few developed sebaceous glands, with a predominance of buds and islands of undifferentiated epithelial cells. The surgeon must remember that the early pathologic impression may not clearly support the clinical diagnosis. As the patient approaches puberty the sebaceous glands become more prominent. At this time appendageal benign tumors (e.g., syringocystadenoma papilliferum) and malignant tumors (basal cell carcinoma) may develop.

SURGICAL TREATMENT

Total excision extending to the clinical margin of the lesion is the acceptable treatment of choice for this particular entity. Excision should extend at least to the depth of hair follicles, which on the scalp are usually to the depth of the superficial to middle subcutaneous fat layer. If the lesion is on the scalp, care must be taken to assess the looseness of scalp tissue when planning primary closure. All borders of the lesion should be checked histopathologically to ensure complete removal because of the pleuripotentiality of these lesions. Excision is recommended before puberty, since the incidence of malignant tumors is increased at this time with the increased proliferation of poorly differentiated cells.

NEUROFIBROMA

CLINICAL DESCRIPTION

Neurofibromas occur in various shapes and sizes. The most common clinical presentation is a soft, sometimes slightly pedunculated lesion, frequently present on the trunk with overlying open comedones on the surface (Fig. 10–10). This lesion has a soft, slightly compressible texture and may sometimes be pushed back into the underlying dermis, the so-called button-hole sign. There may be tremendous variation in size of neurofibromas, ranging from a few millimeters in diameter to several feet in length and diameter.

Although isolated neurofibromas may have no familial predisposition and no associated underlying abnormalities, a search for the familial autosomal dominant neurofibromatosis of von Recklinghausen should be made. Frequently, only a few small neurofibromas may be present on the skin surface and the surgeon may be the first to make the diagnosis of this disease with serious internal and genetic consequences. A search for cafe au lait spots and axillary freckling should be made. Symptomatology referable to almost any system, but especially central nervous and musculoskeletal, may indicate the presence of lesions in critical locations. Characteristic pigment may be found in the eyes by an ophthalmologist. Histopathologic confirmation of neurofibromas should prompt a thorough work-up, including a detailed family history and physical examination, to rule out von Recklinghausen's disease.

HISTOPATHOLOGY FOR THE SURGEON

The important histopathology for the surgeon is that these tumors are not encapsulated and may extend well into the subcutaneous fat.

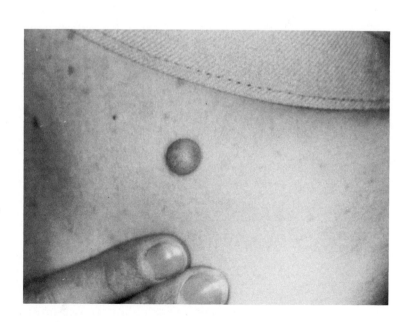

FIGURE 10–10. Neurofibroma.

Some tumors may have a whitish pseudocapsule, but this may be quite adherent to surrounding dermis. A solitary neurofibroma may look pathologically identical to one in a patient with von Recklinghausen's disease, so that other clinical and genetic information must establish that diagnosis for the surgeon.

SURGICAL TREATMENT

Excision is elective and usually done for diagnosis, cosmetic improvement, or release of pressure in a critical area. Complete excision is usually the preferred treatment in such circumstances. One should be aware that underlying deeper extensions and malignant tumors may exist with von Recklinghausen's disease, and one should be prepared for such complications. Excisions should be at least to the subcutaneous tissue level, and histopathologic examination should be done to rule out any extension to deeper tissue. The surgeon should be aware that some lesions (especially in von Recklinghausen's disease) will grow back even more aggressively with partial excision. This factor must be carefully weighed when considering excision of a particular lesion.

If the diagnosis is confirmed and no threat to underlying tissue seems imminent, another cosmetic alternative exists—shave excision. Multiple lesions may be treated quickly and easily in this fashion. Clear documentation of the site of removal should be done for future reference if signs or symptoms of deep invasion develop.

DERMATOFIBROMA

CLINICAL DESCRIPTION

Dermatofibromas are usually poorly defined dermal lesions that appear flesh-colored to an occasional brown color and occur frequently on the extremities (Fig. 10–11). Etiology is usually undetermined, although it is thought that in some circumstances these lesions may follow local trauma. If the skin surrounding a dermatofibroma is pinched, there is a puckering effect created, said to be diagnostic of dermatofibromas. Since the lesion is usually dermal and does not have a capsule or well-defined margin, the diagnosis cannot be completely assured on clinical observation alone.

Lesions may grow slowly over a period of time but usually remain stable in size. They may also acquire a slightly darker pigment with the passage of time.

HISTOPATHOLOGY FOR THE SURGEON

A dermatofibroma is a nonencapsulated tumor of fibroblastic origin. The surgeon should be aware of downward proliferations of the epidermis above these dermal tumors, simulating basal cell carcinoma. True basal cell carcinoma has also been reported with this tumor. Dermatofibrosarcoma protuberans has little chance of being misdiagnosed as a benign dermatofibroma by a good pathologist.

SURGICAL TREATMENT

Excision is my preferred treatment for dermatofibromas. It should be carried to at least the depth of superficial subcutaneous tissue (Fig. 10–11B and C). Pathologic examination of tissue is always made to rule out sarcoma or dermatofibrosarcoma protuberans, although these should

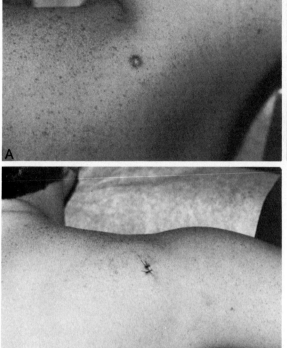

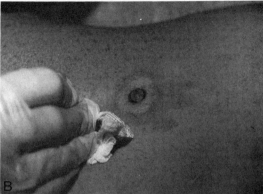

FIGURE 10–11. *A*, Dermatofibroma on upper shoulder. *B*, Circular punch excision. *C*, Closure with two 5–0 nylon sutures.

usually be suspected on clinical grounds. Because the diagnosis may not be made definitively without pathologic examination, methods of removal that do not involve taking a pathologic specimen are preferably not used for these particular lesions.

LEIOMYOMAS

CLINICAL DESCRIPTION

Leiomyomas are usually poorly defined flesh-colored to yellowish or brown lesions frequently appearing on the trunk or extremities. They are often tender or spontaneously painful and may be single or multiple. These lesions may become more numerous with time. Excision of at least one lesion for adequate histopathologic examination should always be done.

HISTOPATHOLOGY FOR THE SURGEON

These nonencapsulated tumors are composed of smooth muscle fibers that can be identified with Masson's trichrome stain. Muscle stains red and collagen green with this stain. If these stains are not used (e.g., the surgeon does not inform the pathologist of a possible leiomyoma), the diagnosis could be missed.

SURGICAL TREATMENT

Complete excision of at least one of these lesions should be done for accurate histopathologic examination. Because these smooth muscle tumors may cause significant pain, if the number of lesions can be approached reasonably with surgical excision, removal of all existing lesions may be carried out. Removal of dozens of small skin tumors at one session is quite easily accomplished. It seems almost incredible that such a procedure is sometimes discussed as being either difficult or perhaps associated with significant morbidity. This should clearly not be the case. If they are asymptomatic and there is no suspicion of malignant degeneration, they may be left untreated. As with most tumors located in the dermis, superficial destructive methods will usually not give the best cosmetic results or provide complete removal of the lesion.

PILOMATRICOMA (CALCIFYING EPITHELIOMA OF MALHERBE)

CLINICAL DESCRIPTION

This tumor usually presents as a single nodule during childhood or early adult life. The skin above it may be flesh colored or have a bluish tinge. It is usually asymptomatic and is found more frequently on the head, neck, and upper extremities. The etiology of this tumor is unknown.

HISTOPATHOLOGY FOR THE SURGEON

This tumor may or may not be encapsulated. It consists essentially of a cellular stroma, shadow cells, and varying amounts of calcium. Calcium may be identified more easily with von Kossa's stain. Bone formation may also be seen in some lesions.

SURGICAL TREATMENT

Surgical treatment of pilomatricoma should be complete excision extending to the level of subcutaneous tissue. Complete excision of all calcified material surrounding the pilomatricoma should be done and carefully assessed at the time of surgery. Destructive methods such as cryosurgery or electrosurgery usually will not adequately remove calcified material in this tumor. Because diagnosis cannot be made with 100 per cent accuracy on clinical observation alone, complete excision with pathologic examination is the treatment of choice.

CYLINDROMA

CLINICAL DESCRIPTION

These lesions are usually found on the scalp as smooth, elevated nodules. When multiple, they frequently have been inherited in an autosomal fashion and increase in number with age. The first lesions will frequently be seen during teen-age years. Numbers may increase dramatically to form the so-called turban-type tumor with almost complete involvement of the scalp surface area; however, in many patients only two or three lesions may exist and these may be removed with excellent cosmetic results. There are rare reports in the literature of malignant degeneration of cylindromas, with most lesions following a totally benign course. When multiple lesions are inherited, multiple trichoepitheliomas (usually on the face) are also common.

HISTOPATHOLOGY FOR THE SURGEON

This tumor consists essentially of islands of epithelial cells surrounded by a hyaline sheath. Glandular lumina may also be found within the tumor. Pathologic diagnosis should be relatively straightforward.

SURGICAL TREATMENT

If the number of lesions is reasonably small, complete surgical excision with primary closure is an acceptable cosmetic and diagnostic procedure. Removal of at least one lesion should always be done for pathologic diagnosis. These lesions are associated with multiple trichoepitheliomas in some families and inherited in an autosomal dominant fashion. One such patient we follow has intermittent removal of only large cylindromas of the scalp causing cosmetic deformity. The patient also has excision, shave removal, and dermabrasion done for many trichoepitheliomas on the face.

TRICHOEPITHELIOMAS

CLINICAL DESCRIPTION

Trichoepitheliomas usually present as flesh-colored to yellowish, slightly elevated papules usually one to several millimeters in diameter. These lesions usually occur on the face, with the nasolabial fold and upper lip perhaps being the most common site of occurrence. There is frequently an autosomal dominant pattern of inheritance with these alone or combined with cylindromas. Lesions will tend to increase in number over time. Clinically, these lesions present a broad differential diagnosis of flesh-colored papules on the face, a few of such differential diagnostic possibilities being syringoma, eccrine spiradenoma, and trichilemmoma associated with breast malignancy (Cowden's disease).

HISTOPATHOLOGY FOR THE SURGEON

The surgeon should be aware of two pitfalls histopathologically. The horn cysts of trichoepithelioma show complete keratinization and should not be confused with the less differentiated horn pearls of squamous cell carcinoma. The total histologic picture makes this unlikely. Keratotic type basal cell carcinoma can closely resemble trichoepithelioma. The surgeon should differentiate solitary or multiple basal cell carcinoma from trichoepithelioma clinically if possible and provide the pathologist with this information.

SURGICAL TREATMENT

There are many acceptable methods with good cosmetic results for removal of trichoepitheliomas. The majority of lesions lie within a limited area on the face. Excision may be a good method for removal of these lesions; however, since they do tend to recur, they may be multiple, and new ones tend to develop over a period of time, care must be taken to conserve tissue.

Superficial dermabrasion or shave excision flush with the surface, followed by light cautery or a styptic agent, gives superior cosmetic results in many cases (Fig. 10–12). It is best to choose a small area to treat before using any surgical method extensively. The surgeon may

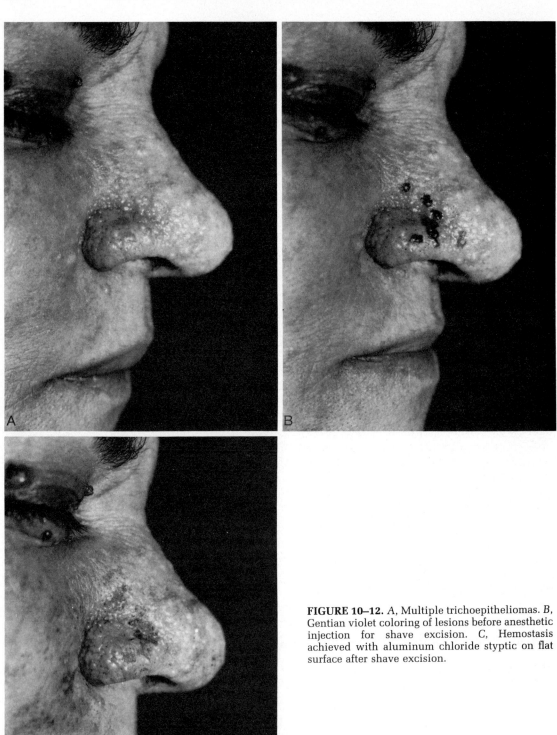

FIGURE 10–12. *A,* Multiple trichoepitheliomas. *B,* Gentian violet coloring of lesions before anesthetic injection for shave excision. *C,* Hemostasis achieved with aluminum chloride styptic on flat surface after shave excision.

then decide which method is most acceptable. Electrosurgery and cry-osurgery are alternative treatments for these lesions.

SYRINGOMAS

CLINICAL DESCRIPTION

Syringomas are flesh-colored to yellow small papules frequently occurring in large numbers on the face. They may also be present on the upper torso and extremities. The periorbital area is especially prone to development of syringomas (Fig. 10–13). Lesions may be confused with many other small, flesh-colored papules, as discussed in the differential diagnosis under trichoepitheliomas.

Syringomas may also be inherited and are seen more frequently in females. When seen in the periorbital area, they may present a differential diagnostic problem with xanthelasma.

HISTOPATHOLOGY FOR THE SURGEON

The strands of epithelial cells, multiple ductal structures, and epithelial cells forming tail-like projections from some of these ducts make histopathologic identification easy in most circumstances. Some mixed adnexal tumors, however, may show some features of these eccrine-derived growths.

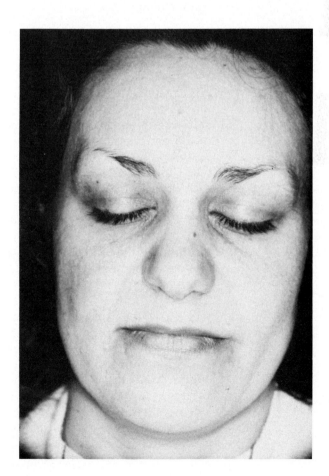

FIGURE 10–13. Periorbital syringomas.

SURGICAL TREATMENT

Treatment of syringomas is usually done for cosmetic reasons. Perhaps the most difficult location is the periorbital region. In this area a syringoma occupies much of the dermis, which is already very thin. Superficial dermabrasion may be done, but only with great caution and skill. Deep abrasion in this area may lead to scarring.

Superficial shaving with light electrodesiccation and aluminum chloride styptic is also a possibility. At times desiccation can precede light curettage for removal of the bulk of the syringoma. An attempt to remove the entire lesion with superficial abrasive methods may lead to unacceptable scarring. Excellent cosmetic results may be obtained by simply removing the elevated portion of the syringoma. Laser treatment may also be successful for small lesions.

If the area is limited, excision may be done, but frequently the extent of involvement precludes surgical excision. If lesions are present on the sternal area, little can be done except for trials of superficial destructive methods. Because of the tendency for scarring in this area, it may be best to leave lesions untreated. Multiple syringomas present a difficult challenge to even the most talented surgeon.

If several methods (electrodesiccation, scalpel shaving, cryosurgery, punch excision, laser therapy, etc.) are tried on one or two lesions in the same patient, one method may show superiority over another for that individual. This approach should be considered with multiple lesions of any type.

XANTHELASMA

CLINICAL DESCRIPTION

Xanthelasma represents a collection of lipid-laden histiocytes in the middle to upper dermis. These lesions are usually of a yellowish or yellowish-orange color and frequently present as flat, plaque-type lesions in the periorbital area. They may or may not be associated with underlying lipoprotein abnormalities. Although they may be present in those with lipoprotein abnormalities early in life, they are more frequently seen in the fourth and fifth decades and later.

HISTOPATHOLOGY FOR THE SURGEON

The essential pathologic feature for the surgeon is the superficial location of the lipid-laden histiocytes in the upper dermis. Surgical treatment need not penetrate to deep dermis or fat in most patients.

SURGICAL TREATMENT

Treatment of xanthelasma is cosmetic. When attempting any surgical treatment, it should be remembered that these represent a collection of histiocytes in the upper or mid-dermis.

If the lesions are limited and can be easily excised, excision is one option. Suturing should be done with a 6-0 nonabsorbable suture and sutures removed at three days with subsequent optional taping. This will give excellent results with xanthelasma of limited extent.

When these lesions involve a larger or strategically difficult area, necessitating grafting, one may consider superficial destructive methods first. Applications of increasing concentrations of trichloroacetic acid may significantly lighten the yellowish or orangish plaques to a point that they are barely perceptible (Fig. 10–14A and B). It is advised that the operator start with a 20 per cent solution of trichloroacetic acid and work up to as high as a 50 per cent solution. This solution is applied to the skin for approximately 20 to 30 seconds or until the skin turns white. Application and removal should be done with small moist cotton-tipped applicators, with care taken never to have any drops of acid drip into the eye. The cotton-tipped applicator is always dabbed on gauze first to remove excess acid. An application of a corticosteroid ointment or cream to the surrounding area may also be used to decrease erythema and any running of minute acid droplets. No taping or special postoperative care is usually necessary. The operator will frequently be amazed at the excellent cosmetic results obtained with weekly or bi-weekly trichloro-acetic acid applications (Fig. 10–14C).

Superficial light electrodesiccation may also be used. Electrodes-iccation followed by light curettage removes the xanthelasma easily (Fig. 10–14D to G). Then very light electrodesiccation may be repeated to shrink the superficial defect left behind. Gentle cleansing of the resulting scab may be done until it falls off. Light pinkish scars usually result in barely perceptible areas within weeks.

Cryosurgery may also be used, but extra care should be exercised since the periorbital dermis is quite thin.

SEBACEOUS HYPERPLASIA

CLINICAL DESCRIPTION

Multiple yellowish papules appearing mostly on the face with increasing age are characteristic of sebaceous hyperplasias. These lesions represent hyperplasia of sebaceous glands surrounding a hair follicle. Examined closely under proper light and magnification, these lesions will be seen to have a central punctum where the follicular orifice exists, surrounded by a lobulated or mulberry-type accumulation of yellowish sebaceous glands.

If these lesions are located in a facial area where superficial blood vessels and telangiectatic vessels exist, stretching of the skin with these elevated papules (as with any elevated lesion of the face) will accentuate the telangiectatic vessel. This will frequently give the lesion an appearance similar to that of basal cell carcinoma. The central punctum is not an ulcerated area, as with the rodent ulcer of basal cell carcinoma. The lobulated yellowish hyperplastic sebaceous glands do not resemble the pearly border of basal cell carcinoma when examined closely. With sebaceous hyperplasias, many lesions of usually the same general size may be found scattered over the entire facial surface, with none of them having ulceration or other characteristic signs of malignancy. If any suspicion exists, biopsy should be done.

These lesions will occur in increasing numbers with age and almost invariably are associated with oily skin. They are usually only a cosmetic problem.

HISTOPATHOLOGY FOR THE SURGEON

The only pathologic finding is hyperplastic sebaceous glands leading to a central follicular duct. No difficulty arises in differentiating this growth from basal cell epithelioma or sebaceous epithelioma.

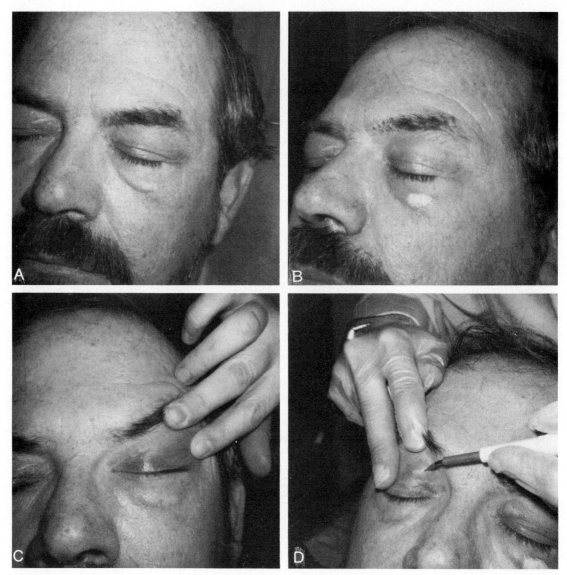

FIGURE 10–14. *A*, Xanthelasma below left eye and on right upper eyelid. *B*, Application of 35 per cent trichloroacetic acid to lesion under left eye causes immediate whitening of the skin. *C*, Slight hypopigmentation left at four weeks after treatment with trichloroacetic acid. *D*, Light electrodesiccation of xanthelasma of right upper eyelid.

Illustration continued on opposite page

SURGICAL TREATMENT

Surgical treatment of these lesions usually involves superficial destructive methods because of the large numbers and small diameter. If only a few lesions exist, excision may be done with either a scalpel or a circular punch. For multiple lesions, either electrodesiccation and light curettage or cryosurgery is the most acceptable form of therapy.

As with any multiple facial lesions where different surgical modalities are acceptable, it is frequently preferable to try a method on one

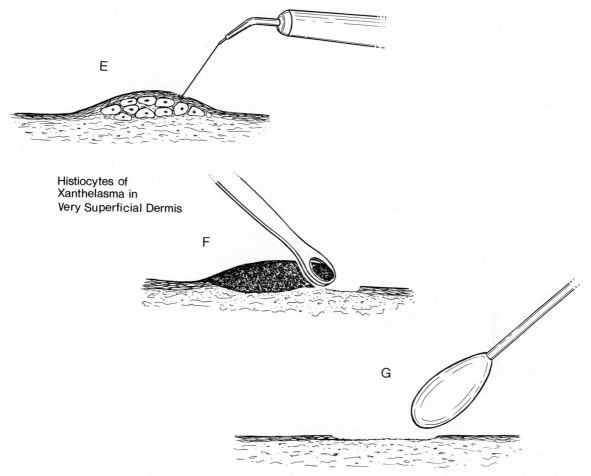

Figure 10–14. *Continued. E* and *F*, Light electrodesiccation of superficial histiocytes of xanthelasma followed by light styptic (*G*).

or two areas prior to treating all existing lesions. Cryotherapy with liquid nitrogen or carbon dioxide often leaves superior cosmetic results. Brief freezing is followed by a small scab that falls off.

Another excellent method is light electrodesiccation of the hyperplastic sebaceous glands with gentle curettage followed again by light desiccation or application of an aluminum chloride styptic (Fig. 10–15). Healing frequently takes place without any subsequent visible scarring after several weeks.

Because of the abundance of pluripotential appendageal structures in these patients, superficial destructive methods will usually give excellent cosmetic results (Fig. 10–16). Because of the frequency of occurrence and numbers of these lesions, excision should be reserved for large lesions or a localized accumulation of a large number of smaller lesions. It should be mentioned that the new drug for acne, 13-cis-retinoic acid, markedly decreases sebum production. One report (Grekin and Ellis, 1983) showed dramatic clearing of sebaceous hyperplasia in a 65-year-old man, but relapse followed discontinuation of the drug.

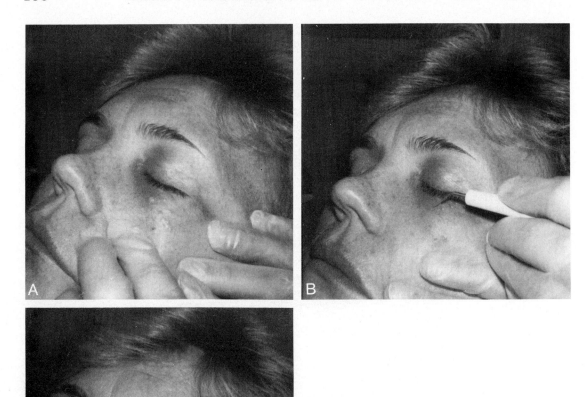

FIGURE 10–15. *A*, Multiple sebaceous hyperplasias. *B*, Light electrocautery with fine epilating-type needle. *C*, Barely perceptible defect resulting.

JUVENILE XANTHOGRANULOMAS

CLINICAL DESCRIPTION

Juvenile xanthogranulomas are usually present in early childhood. These lesions appear clinically as yellowish-orange or orangish-red nodules, plaques, or papules (Fig. 10–17). They may occur anywhere on the skin surface. An examination for eye involvement should be done in patients with juvenile xanthogranulomas.

To the trained practitioner of pediatric dermatology, diagnosis can usually be made without biopsy. Any question as to the diagnosis should prompt biopsy for histopathologic examination. Since these lesions frequently resolve spontaneously without visible scar, surgical treatment is not recommended in most cases. If the lesion is encroaching upon the eye or other functional areas, removal may be necessary. If a single lesion seems to be growing rapidly, excision may be elected.

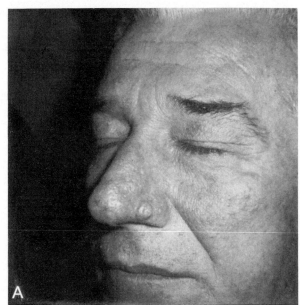

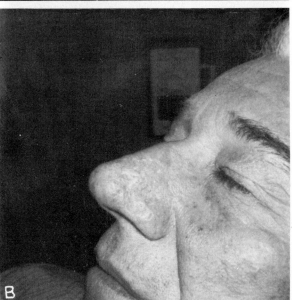

FIGURE 10–16. *A*, Very large sebaceous hyperplasia proven by biopsy. *B*, Four weeks after surgery. Result from shave biopsy and light electrodesiccation.

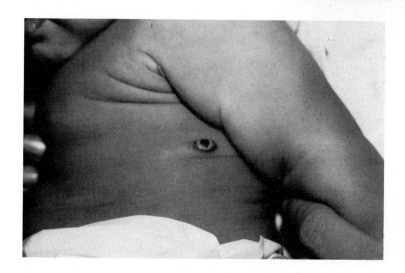

FIGURE 10–17. Juvenile xanthogranuloma.

131

HISTOPATHOLOGY FOR THE SURGEON

Lipid-laden histiocytes and foreign body giant cells with nuclei arranged in a ring-like pattern are characteristic of this lesion. As the lesions resolve, fibrosis may be seen. Clinical and histologic criteria should differentiate xanthogranulomas from histiocytosis syndromes.

SURGICAL TREATMENT

Spontaneous resolution within one to several years is common. Surgical excision is limited to rapidly enlarging lesions encroaching upon vital structures and even in these circumstances may frequently be avoided. If superficial fibrosis is left behind, cosmetic repair can be done at that time.

STRAWBERRY HEMANGIOMAS

CLINICAL DESCRIPTION

These capillary-type hemangiomas are usually present in the first two months of life (Fig. 10–18). An indication for surgical treatment is rapid enlargement encroaching upon vital structures. These lesions will usually resolve spontaneously over a period of several months to several years with adequate cosmetic results.

HISTOPATHOLOGY FOR THE SURGEON

Proliferating endothelial cells and capillary lumina are seen. Fibrosis frequently occurs as the lesion resolves.

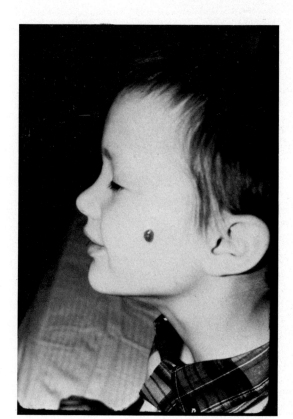

FIGURE 10–18. Strawberry hemangioma.

SURGICAL TREATMENT

Many physicians staunchly believe that no treatment is necessary except in extreme cases of rapidly deforming growth. As an alternative to complex surgical excision, oral prednisone up to 2 mg/kg/day has been used with success by some.

Cryosurgery has also been a favorite for reducing size or stimulating regression. A quick freeze will frequently cause small lesions to crust and fall off.

CAPILLARY HEMANGIOMAS (SENILE ANGIOMAS)

CLINICAL DESCRIPTION

Mature capillary-type angiomas appear with increasing frequency with age. They may first be seen in the third or fourth decade. They usually present as smooth, small, slightly elevated reddish or burgundy-colored papules. They are most frequently located on the trunk, often in large numbers.

The physician should be thoroughly acquainted with the clinical stigmata of angiokeratomas of Fabry's disease. Such lesions show lipid deposits with special staining or electron microscopy and are associated with multiple internal abnormalities. This syndrome should not be confused with benign multiple capillary hemangiomas.

HISTOPATHOLOGY FOR THE SURGEON

A mature capillary-type angioma is seen in the dermis.

SURGICAL TREATMENT

Excision with a circular punch or scalpel can be performed for either cosmetic or diagnostic purposes. It is not necessary to remove all these lesions, and only suspicious or esthetically unacceptable lesions should be removed. Superficial destructive methods may be used if the diagnosis is established. Both electrosurgery and cryosurgery produce good results and are much more acceptable for multiple lesions (Fig. 10–19).

PYOGENIC GRANULOMA

CLINICAL DESCRIPTION

The pyogenic granuloma is actually a capillary-type hemangioma frequently associated with previous trauma. It is usually seen in the young adult population, frequently on the fingers, gingiva, and other areas exposed to trauma.

The lesion is not pyogenic and has no characteristics of a granuloma. The name is an obvious misnomer but has remained. These lesions usually present as rapidly enlarging reddish nodules that achieve maximum size within a period of several weeks. They usually have a slightly oozing granular surface and, therefore, patients frequently seek medical consultation early in their course. There is a slightly increased tendency to develop these lesions during pregnancy.

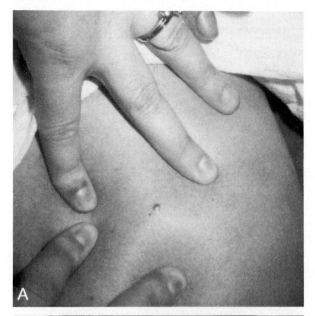

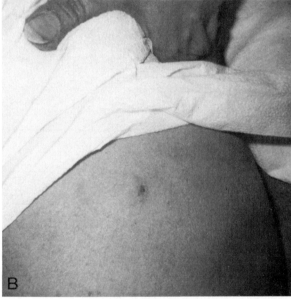

FIGURE 10–19. *A*, Capillary hemangioma. (Note that a small hole from a lidocaine injection can also be seen.) *B*, Light superficial electrodesiccation eradicates the lesion effectively.

HISTOPATHOLOGY FOR THE SURGEON

Multiple endothelial cells in strands and capillary lumina are aggregated close to the epidermis. The epidermis tends to surround the lesion like a collar, accounting for the clinical appearance. This feature is important in classifying the lesion as a pyogenic granuloma.

SURGICAL TREATMENT

If the pyogenic granuloma is located in an area where excision will not compromise valuable tissue, excision is the method of choice. Excision need extend only to the deep dermis.

If the lesion is present in the periungual area or another area where tissue conservation is of utmost importance, electrosurgery or

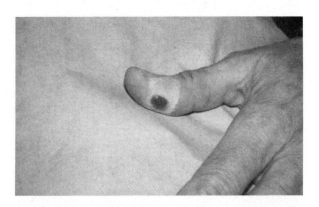

FIGURE 10–20. Pyogenic granuloma. This lesion was easily removed and biopsied with scalpel shave and electrodesiccation. Healing and cosmetic results were excellent.

cryosurgery may be used. Cryosurgery, however, may be difficult in areas such as the finger because of the unpredictable extent of necrosis and possible neuritis. Curettage and electrodesiccation are adequate for removal of these lesions, and less tissue may be compromised. The curette should remove the majority of the lesion intact for histopathologic exam before electrodesiccation is done. Care should be taken not to destroy too much tissue. Removal need be only to the extent of clinical borders (Fig. 10–20).

ANGIOKERATOMA

CLINICAL DESCRIPTION

Angiokeratomas present as round, elevated, purplish papules or nodules (Fig. 10–21). They may be seen associated with the generalized systemic disorder of Fabry's disease or may be seen with increasing age, especially on the scrotum of males. These lesions are benign and are removed for either diagnostic or cosmetic purposes.

HISTOPATHOLOGY FOR THE SURGEON

Most variants of angiokeratoma show dilated capillaries projecting into or surrounded by a thickened epidermis. Special lipid stains and electron microscopy are needed to detect deposits in endothelial cells characteristic of angiokeratoma corporis diffusum (Fabry's disease). The clinical suspicion should be pointed out to the pathologist so that the diagnosis can be confirmed with special studies.

SURGICAL TREATMENT

Complete excision with either a punch or a scalpel is an acceptable method for these small angiomas. These lesions may also be treated with superficial destructive methods (such as cryosurgery or electrosurgery).

DIFFICULT DERMAL AND SUBCUTANEOUS SKIN LESIONS

Any lesion with possible penetration beyond the subcutaneous fat layer or associated underlying deeper abnormalities should not usually be considered suitable for office surgery.

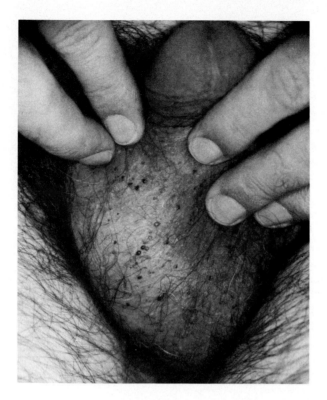

FIGURE 10–21. Angiokeratomas of the scrotum.

Lymphangiomas may appear as well-localized colorless or yellowish blebs on the surface. Clinically, they may appear easy to remove by excisional surgery. These lesions frequently have deeper extensions and also underlying associated abnormalities of the lymphatic and arteriovenous systems.

Lesions lying close to or over the spinal column, and especially those present since birth, could be associated with communications to the spinal canal or underlying abnormalities of the spinal cord. Although these lesions may appear benign and well localized on the surface (especially lipomas), the surgeon should be prepared for possible exploration of the spinal canal.

Large neurofibromas in von Recklinghausen's disease can penetrate deep structures (spinal column, deep nerves, viscera, etc.), and should be approached with caution.

REFERENCES

Arons, M. S., and Hurwitz, S.: Congenital nevocellular nevus: A review of the treatment controversy and a report of 46 cases. Plast. Reconstr. Surg., 72:355, 1983.

Grekin, R. C., and Ellis, C. N.: Report of National Clinical Dermatology Conference. Skin and Allergy News, September, 1983.

Rhodes, A. R., Sober, A. J., Day, C. L., Melski, J. W., Harrist, T. J., Mihm, M. C., Jr., and Fitzpatrick, T. B.: The malignant potential of small congenital nevocellular nevi: An estimate of association based on a histologic study of 234 primary cutaneous melanomas. J. Am. Acad. Dermatol., 6:230, 1982.

chapter 11

BENIGN CYSTIC
SKIN LESIONS

EPIDERMAL CYST

CLINICAL DESCRIPTION

By far the most common cystic lesion seen in the skin is the epidermal cyst. A misunderstanding of its histopathology has led some to call it a sebaceous or oily cyst. This lesion usually presents as a round to oval, whitish to grayish-colored cystic lesion occupying the dermis of the skin. These lesions almost invariably have a central, dark opening that represents the point of invagination of epidermis into a cystic cavity. If the surrounding cyst is firmly squeezed, one can frequently extrude the odoriferous "cheesy" keratinous material characteristic of this cyst.

Often, it is not possible to extrude the keratinous material, but the central opening will be accentuated with firm pressure on the cyst. This opening will usually be of a grayish or grayish-black color. Such a maneuver by the experienced physician almost assures the diagnosis of epidermal cysts (Fig. 11–1).

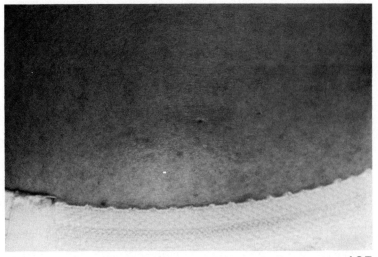

FIGURE 11–1. Dark central opening of an otherwise poorly defined epidermal cyst on the trunk.

Epidermal cysts are seen most frequently on the face, scalp, and trunk areas. The area behind the ear is particularly predisposed. The lesions may be present at any age, usually occurring with increasing frequency after puberty. With the passage of time, many of these lesions will either decrease or increase in size, some of them becoming golf ball size or larger.

It is very common for these lesions to rupture and become inflamed and infected. When this happens, the lesion frequently enlarges significantly. This expansion and pus formation can cause a permanent defect of surrounding skin, making the eventual surgical procedure more extensive and less esthetically acceptable. For these reasons, it is often recommended that such cysts be excised surgically.

HISTOPATHOLOGY FOR THE SURGEON

The essential pathologic features to confirm the diagnosis are the keratinous material and the epidermis-lined cyst itself. When the cyst wall has been fragmented by surgery or spontaneous rupture, inflammation, fibrosis, etc., it is best to look for traces of keratin in the dermis. This search may be aided by the use of polarizing light. As mentioned above, no trace of sebaceous glands or sebum will be found.

SURGICAL TREATMENT

Several different methods exist for surgical removal of epidermal cysts. One such method is to excise an ellipse of overlying skin together with the cyst, the ellipse being approximately 50 per cent the diameter of the cyst. The cyst may then be removed quite easily as the ellipse of skin is pulled outward from the skin surface. Dissection with a curved scissors is usually adequate to free the cyst wall from surrounding fibrotic tissue. After a moderate amount of dissection around the cyst wall, one may apply firm but gentle pressure to the surrounding tissue, causing the cyst to literally pop out (Fig. 11–2).

The removal of extra skin may facilitate the closing of existing dead space after the cystic cavity is removed. If the entire cavity formed

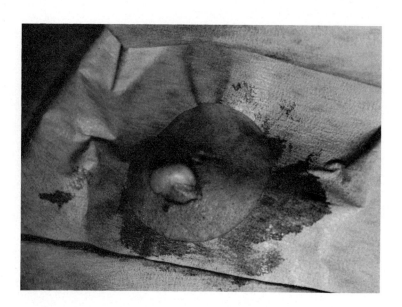

FIGURE 11–2. Epidermal cyst on the jaw has been "popped out" with pressure. Fibrotic attachment to the undersurface of the cyst can be seen.

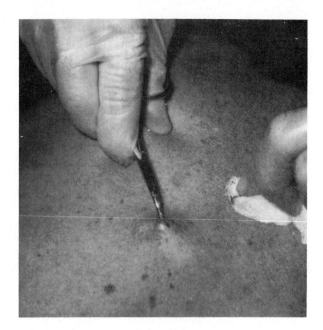

FIGURE 11–3. Grabbing the cyst wall with a hemostat for complete removal.

by compression of the growing cyst is large and is left and sutured over, hematoma and infection may follow. An attempt should be made to obliterate existing dead space.

For epidermal cysts that are small in size or have not had extensive inflammation with subsequent fibrosis, incision and removal of the sack in toto may be done. One method is simply to make a very short midline incision over the central opening of the cyst, and drain all the keratinous debris by firm pressure on all sides. One may then grab the cyst itself with a hemostat or forceps with teeth, extracting the cyst wall in toto (Fig. 11–3). Sometimes this method will necessitate the use of a fine curved iris scissors to dissect some of the cyst wall from surrounding tissue. If there has been significant inflammation with subsequent fibrosis and attachment of the cyst wall to surrounding tissues, this method may be inadequate. The cyst wall must always be removed or the cyst will recur.

An alternative method is to make a small incision over the midline of the cyst without actually puncturing the cyst wall. Frequently, gentle pressure and dissection, as explained above, will allow the cyst to be popped from this small hole by firm pressure on all sides. For small cysts that have not been inflamed previously, this will frequently deliver the cyst from an incision line shorter than the cyst diameter itself. Simple Steri-Strips or one or two sutures will usually close such an incision adequately.

When epidermal cysts are inflamed or infected, an effort should be made to drain as much keratinous material and pus as possible by incision and drainage done at the original external opening of the skin. This should be followed by frequent moist, warm compresses and an antibiotic effective against gram-positive cocci. Antibiotics should be continued for approximately 10 days. It is wise not to excise the cyst until several weeks after inflammation and infection have resolved. Such cysts should preferably be surgically excised, even if the size is reduced considerably. The cyst itself will not disappear or dissolve, and even if clinically undetectable, it remains inactive only temporarily. There is a significant chance of further cosmetic deformity with any subsequent infection and accompanying enlargement of the cyst.

PILAR CYSTS

CLINICAL DESCRIPTION

The pilar cyst is usually located on the scalp and clinically may resemble the epidermal cyst; however, the pilar cyst does not as frequently have a central opening as the epidermal cyst. Nor does the pilar cyst have the tendency to drain keratinous material as frequently as epidermal cysts do. This cyst is seen somewhat more frequently in later years and may be multiple. There may be some familial predisposition to the development of pilar cysts. These cysts do not seem to have the frequent tendency that epidermal cysts have for the development of infection, probably because of the lack of frequent communication with the surface. Because of their size, the cysts usually present a cosmetic problem. They may frequently become very hard because of calcification that often accompanies such cysts.

HISTOPATHOLOGY FOR THE SURGEON

Three pathologic features clearly separate the pilar cyst from the epidermal cyst. (1) The keratinous material in the pilar cyst is rather amorphous compared to the laminated keratin of epidermal cysts. (2) Pilar cyst wall cells are not as clearly demarcated with a progressive keratinization as with epidermal cysts. The wall of the epidermal cyst more closely resembles true epidermis. (3) Calcium deposits are frequently seen in pilar cysts.

SURGICAL TREATMENT

If the pilar cyst is less than 2 cm in diameter, it can frequently be removed with a central incision approximately the diameter of the cyst. Frequently, the cyst may be delivered directly out of this incision by firm pressure on all sides. These cysts are more likely to be removed in toto because the lesser incidence of inflammation and infection leads to fewer fibrous adhesions with surrounding tissue. The cyst wall is very frequently smooth and unattached to surrounding structures. If the cyst is larger than 2 cm, the method of using an elliptical incision approximately 50 per cent the size of the cystic lesion should be employed. Inspection of the cystic cavity after the pilar cyst is removed may lead to the decision of taking even a greater amount of surrounding skin to avoid leaving dead space. One should be careful of removing so much surrounding skin that wound edges cannot be approximated. Many scalps have very little laxity, and closure may be quite difficult. Moving tissue over a convex surface such as the scalp also requires more force and tension than moving the same tissue in a horizontal plane (Fig. 11–4). If undermining is necessary to close the resulting defect, it should be subgaleal, as this area is relatively avascular and only loose areolar tissue needs to be dissected. Further relaxation of scalp may be done by scoring the underlying galea. As with any scalp surgery, manipulation of the scalp should be done before undertaking the operation to determine the laxity of the individual's scalp tissue. This is extremely important

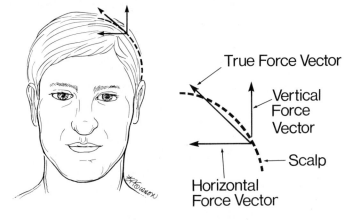

FIGURE 11–4. When approximating wound edges over a convex scalp, both horizontal and vertical forces must be used. The resulting force vector is greater than the horizontal force vector needed to approximate most other wounds.

because of the significant variability of elasticity or laxity of scalp tissue in different individuals and at different ages. Removal of more than 2 cm of scalp tissue may be difficult in some individuals.

APOCRINE HIDROCYSTOMA

CLINICAL DESCRIPTION

These are cystic lesions usually located on the face or less commonly on the trunk area. They frequently have a thin overlying layer of epidermis and dermis and may display a light blue discoloration on clinical examination. The cysts are usually solitary and may occur at any age. Usually clinical examination raises strong suspicion of the diagnosis (Fig. 11–5). There is no familial tendency and lesions do not tend to recur.

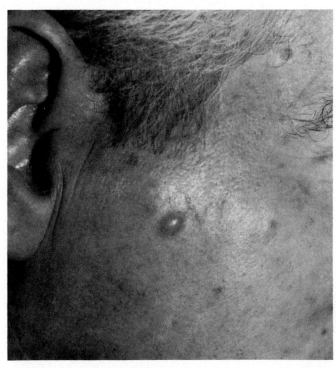

FIGURE 11–5. Apocrine hidrocystoma of the cheek. Excision confirmed clinical suspicion.

HISTOPATHOLOGY FOR THE SURGEON

Pathologic diagnosis is relatively straightforward, with secretory cells lining a well-defined cystic structure. The less common eccrine hidrocystoma could be considered in the differential diagnosis.

SURGICAL TREATMENT

The preferred method of treatment of apocrine hidrocystoma is complete excision. Excision need extend only to the deep dermis or superficial subcutaneous tissue, as lesions are usually limited to the dermis. The entire specimen should be submitted for histopathologic examination. If the lesion is treated early, there is usually excellent cosmetic results with excision. If it is allowed to grow in an area such as the periorbital area, more extensive procedures such as skin grafting may be necessary.

DIGITAL MUCOUS CYSTS

CLINICAL DESCRIPTION

These cysts usually develop suddenly, perhaps in relation to trauma. They are more common in adulthood. There is no evidence of familial inheritance. They usually will not resolve spontaneously. They are most common on the fingers distal to the distal interphalangeal joint (Fig. 11–6).

HISTOPATHOLOGY FOR THE SURGEON

A cystic cavity in the dermis contains mostly mucin that is PAS-negative. It does not usually involve deep structures such as tendon or bone.

SURGICAL TREATMENT

In some cases the cyst will drain mucinous material if punctured and slightly compressed. Since these usually occur in areas with little

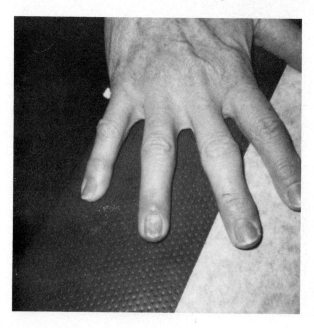

FIGURE 11–6. Digital mucous cyst at proximal nail fold (over matrix) of ring finger. Pressure on the matrix has caused a deep groove (the width of the cyst) in the nail.

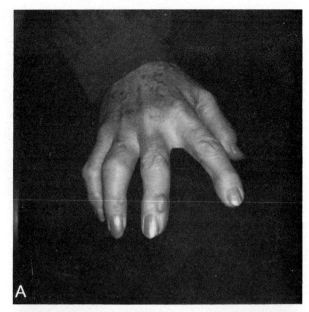

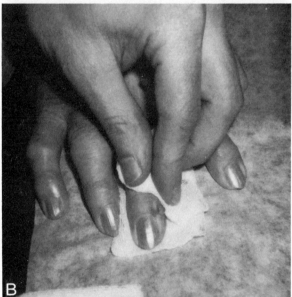

FIGURE 11–7. *A,* Another digital mucous cyst. *B,* Extrusion of thick, completely clear mucinous material diagnostic of digital mucous cyst. The lesion did not recur after complete drainage.

skin to spare, this symptomatic therapy may be the best course of action in some cases (Fig. 11–7).

If pathologic confirmation is needed and the surgeon wishes to avoid complete excision, a small punch biopsy can be done. Of course, if necessary, total excision can be performed.

Some patients will show recurrence of these cysts even after surgical treatment.

ORAL MUCOUS CYSTS

CLINICAL DESCRIPTION

These cysts usually appear suddenly on the lips or buccal mucosa. They usually result from the blockage or rupture of salivary glands (Fig. 11–8).

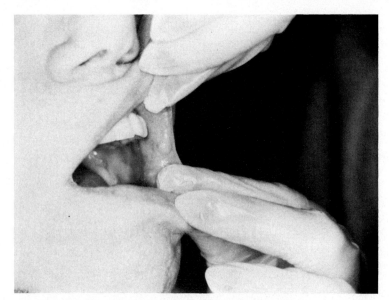

FIGURE 11–8. Oral mucous cyst.

HISTOPATHOLOGY FOR THE SURGEON

These cysts contain mostly sialomucin and stain positive with PAS, in contrast to the digital mucous cyst, which is PAS-negative.

SURGICAL TREATMENT

Simple puncture and drainage are usually adequate. If biopsy confirmation is necessary, removal with the scalpel or circular punch is quite acceptable. Closure is usually with absorbable suture material.

chapter 12

MALIGNANT
SKIN TUMORS

Basal cell carcinoma (rodent ulcer) is the most common malignancy in the United States today. Conservative estimates place the incidence of this tumor at 400,000 per year in the United States.

Clinically, this lesion presents as a slowly growing tumor studded with telangiectases and usually characterized by a pearly border. Frequently, there is central ulceration with continued growth. These lesions are locally destructive but rarely metastasize.

There seems to be a direct correlation between sun exposure over a long period of time and the development of basal cell carcinoma. Evidence to support this theory is the usual location on sun-exposed skin, a higher incidence in light-skinned and blue-eyed individuals, an increased incidence in sunnier climates, and the rare occurrence in black-skinned individuals.

Despite the heavy evidence for sun-induced etiology, certain areas that are exposed to heavy actinic damage over the years, such as the dorsum of the hands, have a very low incidence of basal cell carcinoma. The same areas have a very high rate of actinic keratoses and subsequent squamous cell carcinoma. One theory to explain this apparent discrepancy is that adequate pilosebaceous structures with pluripotential cells provide a more fertile ground for the development of basal cell carcinoma. It still seems probable that basal cell carcinoma is directly sun-induced in many instances, with exceptions, such as the dorsum of the hands, being related to some other unknown factor.

Before attempting to treat a basal cell carcinoma, one should be thoroughly acquainted with the different morphologic clinical types, their different patterns of invasion, and their growth rates. Identification of clinical and histopathologic type will frequently influence the treatment modality to be used.

By far the most common type of basal cell carcinoma is the nodular ulcerative form. This type of basal cell carcinoma has led to the descriptive term "rodent ulcer." There may be central ulceration with surrounding lobulated nodular tumor growth with a pearly border, usually studded with telangiectatic blood vessels most marked at the periphery (Fig.

145

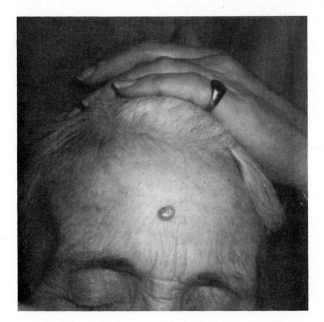

FIGURE 12–1. Nodular basal cell carcinoma with pearly color and studded with telangiectases.

12–1). The diagnosis of such lesions can usually be made with reasonable assurance by the clinical appearance alone. Treatment may frequently proceed at the time of initial biopsy, rather than as a two-stage procedure.

A less common form of basal cell carcinoma is the sclerosing or morphea-like basal cell carcinoma. This usually presents as a poorly outlined yellowish plaque, frequently on the face (Fig. 12–2). Telangiectatic blood vessels are not always as prominent as with nodular ulcerative basal cell carcinoma but may be seen when the skin is stretched. Definition of borders both clinically and histopathologically can be quite difficult with this lesion, leading to a much higher recurrence rate for this subtype of basal cell carcinoma. A thick connective tissue with thin

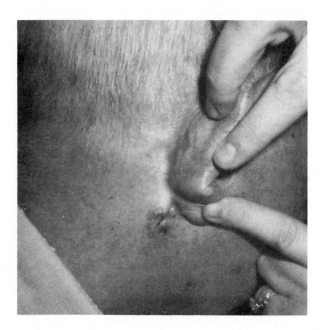

FIGURE 12–2. Sclerosing or morphea-form basal cell carcinoma. Central area is more nodular, but a yellowish plaque is seen extending beyond the nodular area.

strands and islands of basal cell carcinoma histologically correlates well with the clinical identification of finger-like projections extending beyond the gross clinical border.

The least aggressive and slowest growing of the major types of basal cell carcinoma is the superficial basal cell carcinoma. It is possible that different etiologic factors are involved in the development of this particular malignancy. This lesion frequently presents on the trunk in contrast to the predominantly facial location of nodular basal cell carcinomas. It is also more frequently associated with previous arsenic ingestion and the development of arsenical keratoses and Bowen's disease in some patients. This lesion is characterized by a slightly elevated reddish plaque with occasional scaling. It is usually a very slow-growing lesion with a characteristic thready, pearly border at many of the edges (Fig. 12–3). With the use of a hand lens, this border may be seen to have prominent telangiectatic blood vessels. Many of these patients will have had a lesion present for 10 to 20 years or more without any evidence of deep invasion or metastasis. All patients with these lesions should be carefully questioned as to previous arsenic ingestion over the last 20 to 30 years or more (e.g., Fowler's solution, Asiatic pills, contaminated well water, extensive contact with pesticides, or any unknown treatments in the past for psoriasis or atopic dermatitis). These patients should always be followed carefully with or without a positive history of arsenic ingestion for the development of arsenical keratoses (especially on the palms), Bowen's disease, and squamous cell carcinoma.

HISTOPATHOLOGY FOR THE SURGEON

With superficial basal cell carcinoma, small projections of basal cells are seen penetrating superficial dermis only. Most of these still have a noticeable connection to the epidermis. Superficial basal cell carcinoma lacks the multiple islands of basal cells entirely within the dermis that are seen in other types of basal cell carcinoma.

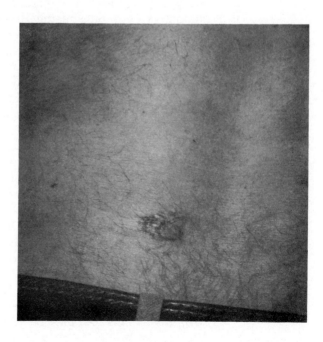

FIGURE 12–3. Superficial and pigmented basal cell carcinoma of the trunk. This patient had five such lesions on the trunk, but none on the face. Previous arsenic exposure was suspected.

Noduloulcerative basal cell carcinoma shows islands of basal cells invading the dermis in most cases. The surgeon should be particularly concerned with any basal cell carcinoma that penetrates beyond the dermis, since this may indicate a particularly aggressive form of basal cell carcinoma. Larger borders and frozen section control would be preferable for such tumors.

Morphea-like or sclerosing basal cell carcinoma is recognized histologically by an increase in fibrous tissue stroma and by thin strands of basal cells. A correlation of this with the clinical characteristics isolate the sclerosing basal cell as a distinct entity. The surgeon must be extremely careful to obtain adequate margins and to have the borders of the excision checked with multiple serial sections.

SURGICAL TREATMENT

After the clinical and pathologic type of basal cell carcinoma has been determined, the treatment may be chosen. The most common forms of treatment for basal cell carcinoma are excisional surgery or curettage and electrodesiccation. Radiation and cryosurgery may also be used but do not provide the physician with a histopathologic specimen or the ability to determine accurately complete removal of the lesion. Microscopically controlled surgery (Mohs' surgery) is a method used usually for recurrent tumors, aggressive or large tumors, or tumors whose recurrence is likely (e.g., morphea-like basal cell carcinoma).

For many basal cell carcinomas excisional surgery offers both superior esthetic results and a complete specimen to check for invasion of the margins. A microscopic check can be done to determine the adequacy of excision. This specimen is not available with radiation, curettage and electrodesiccation, and cryosurgery. Primary closure may give a better esthetic result than letting the wound granulate (as frequently done in Mohs' microscopically controlled surgery).

If the clinical borders are well defined and basal cell carcinoma is less than 2 cm in diameter, a 2- to 5-mm border is usually sufficient. One study of 634 basal cell carcinomas excised by two plastic surgeons compared cure rates using different margins of normal tissue.[1] One surgeon routinely took a 2- to 3-mm border, while the other used margins of grossly normal tissue on all sides at least as wide as the diameter of the tumor. At the end of three years similar cure rates of approximately 98.6 per cent were obtained by both methods. Another study showed that at least one high power field of normal tissue between the specimen edge and the tumor gave an acceptable 10-year recurrence rate (1.2 per cent).[2] In this same study lesions with tumor at the surgical margin showed a 33 per cent recurrence rate. Most studies have also shown that recurrences are most common within the first few years after excision,[3] so that the patient should be followed closely during this period. When excision and primary closure are used, the histopathologic specimen should be examined carefully and uniformly for extension of tumor to the margins of the excised specimen.

In difficult cases where there may be a question concerning tumor extending to the border, I developed another method for more accurately checking the specimen edge.[4] This method involves the use of either one of two special surgical tools. One such method involves the use of parallel scalpels (Taylor double blade) originally used by a surgeon for strip grafts. This tool may be adjusted to cut a specimen 1.5 to 2 mm or

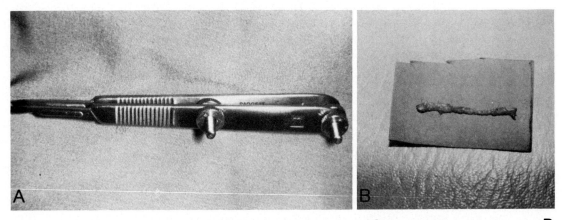

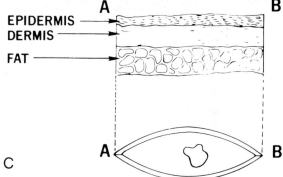

EPIDERMIS
DERMIS
FAT

A   B

A   B

C

FIGURE 12–4. *A,* Taylor double blade. *B,* Strip of tissue removed with Taylor blade. *C,* Schematic of border strip.

more in thickness (Fig. 12–4). With the excision of a routine ellipse, two thin sections representing the entire lateral border of the tumor are obtained. These specimens may be laid flat and cut tangentially to represent the entire border of the tumor. It can be easily seen that no matter how many vertical sections are made, it is always possible to miss tumor extension, since these sections do not represent the entire border of the tumor (Fig. 12–5). This method may also be used in conjunction with a slice of tissue from the bottom of the surgical specimen for

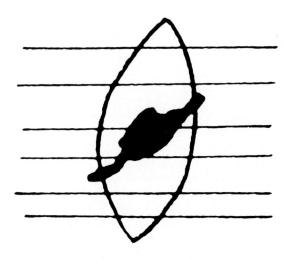

FIGURE 12–5. Vertical sections may miss tumor extension to margins.

evidence of deep extension. Free-hand slices of lateral margins can and are done by surgical pathologists, but this is technically quite difficult on all but large specimens. Special care should be given to examining this specimen if there is any evidence of penetration into subcutaneous tissue with routine vertical sections on the body of the specimen. In most cases penetration to subcutaneous tissue does not occur and this is not a problem.

A second instrument is a circular punch with concentric cutting edges allowing for a 2-mm circular outer specimen to be obtained (Fig. 12–6). The appropriate size punch is selected (the same diameter as would be used in routine elliptical incision). The tumor and surrounding border are first punched with this instrument, with subsequent elliptical excision proceeding as usual. The outer 2-mm piece of tissue is laid flat and cut tangentially for complete examination of the border of the tumor (Fig. 12–7). Again a specimen is taken horizontally from the bottom. This method is much quicker and involves less tissue sectioning than does use of the double scalpel. If surgery is done close to a frozen tissue laboratory, sections may be processed and examined before primary closure. This is usually not necessary for routine basal cell carcinoma. This instrument is also helpful in checking borders when removing a circular piece of tissue for grafting. Processing of the 2-mm strip may be done while the graft is being prepared.

Curettage with electrodesiccation is the most common method used by dermatologists in this country for treatment of basal cell carcinoma. It is a time-honored treatment with cure rates comparable to those of excisional surgery. The healing time is usually two to four weeks or

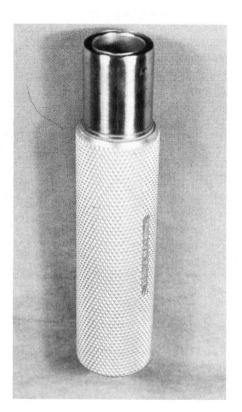

FIGURE 12–6. Double punch with concentric cutting edges.

DOUBLE EDGE CIRCULAR PUNCH

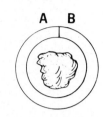

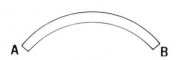

FIGURE 12–7. Circular border obtained is cut between A and B and laid flat for sectioning.

more. With excisional surgery adequate healing can be expected within one to two weeks. For the patient concerned with immediate esthetic results (especially the patient who has had multiple lesions removed over a period of years), excisional surgery may be preferable. It has been argued that the curette may find soft tumor masses in the dermis not detected with the razor-sharp scalpel. In many situations the esthetic result with curettage and electrodesiccation may be superior to that with excision. The frequently shorter but wider scar obtained with curettage and electrodesiccation may be preferable to a longer thin scar of excision in certain instances. This may be true where more extensive surgery with flaps, grafts, or other modifications of incision lines may be necessary for excisional surgery (Figs. 12–8 and 12–9).

One location where curettage with electrodesiccation seems to be esthetically superior to scalpel surgery is on the nose, where a graft is usually required after surgical excision. The scar resulting from curettage and electrodesiccation is usually superior to that of even the best graft. If curettage with electrodesiccation is done in the area of the nasolabial fold, it may result in a sclerotic and sometimes hypertrophic scar studded with telangiectatic blood vessels. This may not leave a cosmetic result as acceptable as that obtained with excisional surgery. In addition, a sclerotic telangiectatic scar may hinder the diagnosis of recurrent basal cell carcinoma because of similarities to the tumor itself; however, a trained eye can usually recognize the difference.

Despite some disadvantages, electrodesiccation with curettage remains a very acceptable and effective treatment for primary nodular basal cell carcinoma. It may be preferable to excision for superficial basal cell carcinoma, since the shallow scar that remains is usually better than a wider excision, perhaps requiring a flap or graft. It should probably not routinely be used for sclerosing basal cell carcinoma, because the curette may lose its ability to distinguish soft tumor from healthy dermis in this fibrous tumor.

Microscopically controlled surgery by Mohs' technique usually involves saucer-shaped excisions of small pieces of tissue. A map is made of the saucerized area and each small piece of tissue stained with a dye for orientation. The small pieces of tissue are flattened and frozen

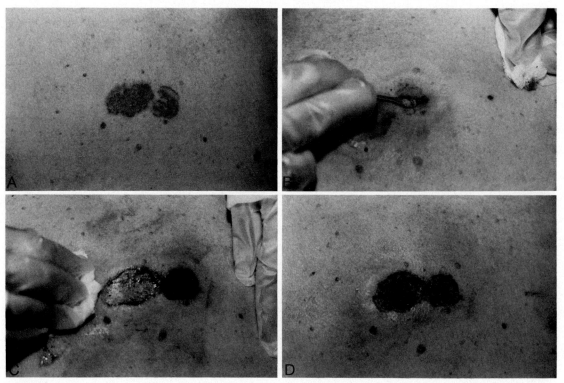

FIGURE 12–8. *A*, Superficial type basal cell carcinoma. *B*, Curettage in the upper dermis easily removed this superficial tumor, with firm dermis (healthy tissue) encountered readily. *C*, Bleeding base after curettage. *D*, Hemostasis achieved.

sections are done. Each section that shows tumor is saucerized again with additional frozen sections until no tumor is detected. The wound is left open to granulate from the edges in, a process usually taking several weeks or more. This method usually gives superior cure rates.[5] (99 per cent or better in certain locations), but may leave wider scars than cosmetically desired in certain circumstances. It is also necessary for the patient to tolerate an undesirable cosmetic appearance during the period of healing. The necessity of a frozen section laboratory and trained personnel also limits the availability of this method. Most surgeons and dermatologists would reserve this method for either recurrent tumors, large tumors, or an area where little normal tissue is available for excisional surgery.

SQUAMOUS CELL CARCINOMA AND BOWEN'S DISEASE

CLINICAL DESCRIPTION

Squamous cell carcinoma is a common tumor occurring in areas of chronic actinic damage, usually presenting as a more indurated lesion in an area of previous actinic keratosis. The sun-exposed areas are primarily involved, with the face, bald scalp, and dorsum of the arms and hands being the most common locations (Fig. 12–10).

A differentiation should be made clinically and histopathologically between squamous cell carcinoma arising from an actinic keratosis and squamous cell carcinoma arising de novo, from burn scars, from mucous

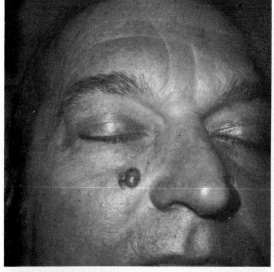
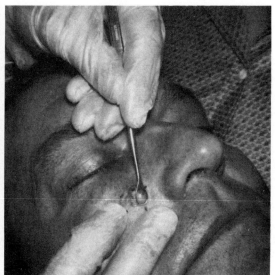
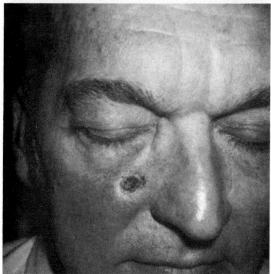

FIGURE 12–9. *A,* Nodular primary basal cell carcinoma. *B,* Removal of lesion with curettage. *C,* Appearance immediately after curettage and electrodesiccation.

membrane surfaces, or from chronic draining sinuses or ulcers. The squamous cell carcinoma arising in areas of actinic damage has an extremely low tendency to metastasize and a very slow growth rate.[6] It is only this type of squamous cell carcinoma that should be approached routinely as office surgery. These lesions are usually seen in the fifth decade or later, and a familial tendency toward actinic damage is usually present. If the patient is followed closely there is little chance of deep invasion or metastases in most patients. Patients who are immunosuppressed, however, may experience rapid metastasis of squamous cell carcinoma in actinic skin. The surgeon should be acutely aware of any such underlying problem.

Bowen's disease is considered by many to be squamous cell carcinoma in situ (limited to the epidermis). This is frequently seen in patients who have had previous arsenic intake, as mentioned under basal cell carcinoma. In any of these patients a careful search of all skin

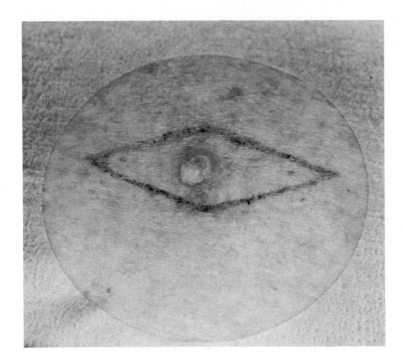

FIGURE 12–10. Typical squamous cell carcinoma arising from an actinic keratosis on sun-damaged skin.

surfaces should be done routinely for other skin cancers such as basal cell carcinoma.

The patient with squamous cell carcinoma arising from an actinic keratosis almost invariably has several other actinic keratoses and will usually develop more in the future. These patients should be followed closely, with actinic keratoses being treated by curettage and electrodesiccation, cryosurgery, or topical 5-fluorouracil. (See section on actinic keratoses.)

HISTOPATHOLOGY FOR THE SURGEON

Perhaps the most important histologic features for the surgeon are those that may classify a squamous cell carcinoma as one arising in an area of actinic damage. Elastotic degeneration of collagen, dysplastic epidermal cells in a haphazard arrangement, and variable hyperkeratosis are clues to actinic damage. If deep invasion is not present, such squamous cell carcinoma is not likely to have metastasized. Conservative excision of the borders of the lesion may be done in this circumstance with good histologic checking of the margins.

Accurate clinical information should alert the pathologist to the possibility of keratoacanthoma or pseudoepitheliomatous hyperplasia in the differential diagnosis. A keratoacanthoma does not require a wide margin of normal tissue, and pseudoepitheliomatous hyperplasia may be a manifestation of many different benign and infectious processes (e.g., gummatous syphilis, blastomycosis, chronic ulcers, etc.).

SURGICAL TREATMENT

If squamous cell carcinoma has developed from actinically damaged skin, a conservative border (3 to 5 mm) is usually sufficient. Careful examination of the specimen should be done to rule out invasion of the surgical borders. Without evidence of deep extension or lymphadenopathy, these lesions may be excised locally without regional node dissection. If there is a question as to the etiology of the squamous cell carcinoma, or particularly bothersome histopathologic features are present, the lesion should be excised with larger margins. Although locally destructive methods such as curettage and electrodesiccation suffice as treatment for early superficial lesions, excision is usually preferred for larger lesions.

KERATOACANTHOMA

CLINICAL DESCRIPTION

The most common form of keratoacanthoma seen by the practicing physician is solitary keratoacanthoma. This lesion usually presents as a rapidly growing tumor, frequently on sun-exposed skin. It usually has a central keratinous crater with a surrounding elevated border, somewhat resembling a volcano (Fig. 12–11). It is sometimes difficult to differentiate this lesion clinically from a rapidly growing squamous cell carcinoma. The lesion frequently reaches a size of 2 cm or more within several weeks.

HISTOPATHOLOGY FOR THE SURGEON

The surgical specimen must be wide enough to include a complete margin and must penetrate the complete depth of the dermis. The

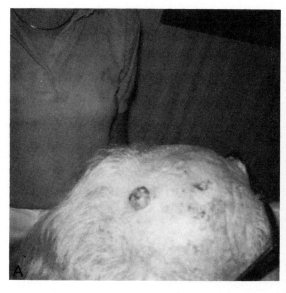

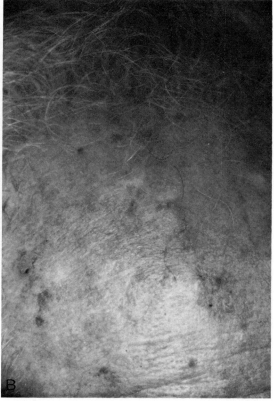

FIGURE 12–11. A, Solitary keratoacanthoma on the scalp of a patient with extensive actinic damage. The lesion developed rapidly over three weeks' time. B, Smooth flat white scar four weeks after deep shave and electrodesiccation. No recurrence at one year.

buttressing so characteristic of this tumor is seen at the edges, with a central crater of keratinous material. Dermal invasion is relatively uniform as one scans the slide from one lateral border to the other. The irregular deep invasion seen with squamous cell carcinoma is usually absent.

SURGICAL TREATMENT

Complete excision is an acceptable method for removal of this lesion and is favored for the following reasons: (1) A complete surgical specimen guarantees a more accurate histopathologic diagnosis, with the characteristic buttressing seen at the tumor margins. (2) The lesion may continue to enlarge rapidly, causing more tissue destruction that eventuates in a larger scar. (3) The cosmetic result from surgical excision is usually distinctly superior to the scar left after occasional spontaneous involution of the lesion. (4) Squamous cell carcinoma is sometimes a possibility even with careful histologic examination. Tumor margins should be adequate to ensure complete removal of the lesion and should extend to the depth of subcutaneous tissue. Any question as to the involvement of tumor edges should prompt excision of additional tissue.

DERMATOFIBROSARCOMA PROTUBERANS

CLINICAL DESCRIPTION

Dermatofibrosarcoma protuberans begins as an area of induration with irregular borders frequently occurring on the trunk (Fig. 12–12). It may be very poorly defined, and a pathologic specimen is necessary for diagnosis. This is a slowly growing tumor that usually is limited to dermis and subcutaneous tissue at the clinical onset. However, it is notorious for extension beyond clinically visible and palpable borders, with invasion frequently occurring in deep dermis or subcutaneous tissue laterally. Metastases have been reported to occur and were present in 5 of 86 cases in one report.[7]

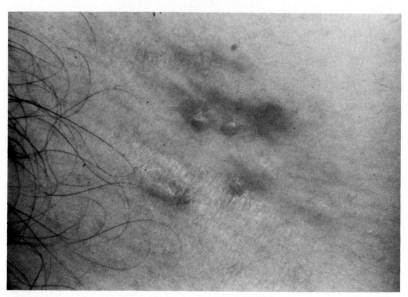

FIGURE 12–12. Dermatofibrosarcoma protuberans. (Photo courtesy of James B. Pinski, M.D.)

HISTOPATHOLOGY FOR THE SURGEON

As mentioned above, this tumor is notorious for lateral extension beyond clinical margins. The pathologist should be urged to examine completely all clinical borders. The use of the variable width knife (discussed under Basal Cell Carcinoma) by the surgeon to take 2-mm strips of the outer margins at surgery may facilitate histopathologic checking.[4] These strips may be mounted as flat sections representing the entire tumor border. It is also advisable to excise fascia and even examine muscle for invasion by this slowly aggressive tumor. Very close clinical follow-up with quick biopsy of any new suspicious areas should be done.

SURGICAL TREATMENT

Excision should always include a very wide margin and deep fascia. As mentioned above, muscle excision for histopathologic checking is also helpful. There are at least two reports of successful management with Mohs' microscopically controlled surgery.

PAGET'S DISEASE

CLINICAL DESCRIPTION

This lesion is mentioned simply to remind the reader of the extent of associated underlying malignancy with Paget's disease either of the breast or of the extramammary region. This lesion usually presents as a scaling red plaque that has been resistant to all forms of topical therapy (Fig. 12–13). When present in the nipple area it is almost invariably associated with underlying intraductal carcinoma of the breast. When present in the groin and perianal area it is frequently associated with underlying apocrine gland carcinoma or rectal carcinoma.

HISTOPATHOLOGY FOR THE SURGEON

With extramammary Paget's disease careful serial sectioning must be done to detect any carcinoma of apocrine or eccrine glands. Also, there is a higher incidence of associated adenocarcinoma of the rectum with Paget's disease in the perianal region.

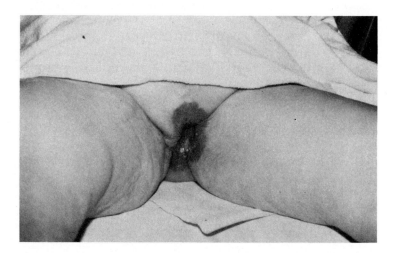

FIGURE 12–13. Extramammary Paget's disease.

SURGICAL TREATMENT

Wide excision plus a search for associated underlying carcinoma is the treatment of choice. It should be pointed out that microscopically controlled surgery in the past has identified Paget's disease several centimeters beyond the clinical border.[8] This should be considered when recommending surgery for such patients.

MELANOMA

It is beyond the scope of this book to discuss the surgical treatment of malignant melanoma. We would simply like to mention the proper method of obtaining a biopsy for a lesion suspicious of melanoma. Although there has been no direct evidence that tumor is spread by incisional biopsy through the tumor, most surgeons prefer a complete excisional biopsy where at all feasible. This not only avoids the theoretical possibility of spreading tumor with the scalpel but also allows for an accurate histopathologic determination of the type, level, and thickness of the tumor—important factors in determining the type and extent of surgical treatment. In addition, any suspicious lesion should be sectioned throughout the entire lesion, since malignancy may be present in only one small portion and tumor thickness may vary. If possible, a 3- to 5-mm border extending to the depth of subcutaneous tissue or superficial fascia should be included in the excision for biopsy of highly suspicious lesions.

Careful, accurate measurement should be made of all borders before excision is done. These measurements should be recorded on the patient's chart. This is for the benefit of the surgeon who will do a wider excision if the lesion proves to be a malignant melanoma. It is also preferable when possible to orient the excisional biopsy in the direction of lymphatic flow. This may be the direction of further excision if melanoma is found.

KAPOSI'S SARCOMA

CLINICAL DESCRIPTION

Kaposi's sarcoma usually presents as purple, red, or brownish papules or nodules, frequently seen over the lower extremities. The type of Kaposi's sarcoma seen in the United States usually presents after the fourth or fifth decade and tends to be slowly growing. This seems to be a truly multicentric tumor, with multiple nodules representing multiple primary lesions, rather than metastatic lesions. This factor influences treatment in many localized cases. The upper extremities are the second most common area of occurrence in the skin, with the gastrointestinal tract being the most likely area for internal involvement. For more complete discussion of this multicentric tumor the reader should refer to dermatology text books or a monograph on the subject by Bluefarb.[9]

More recently, Kaposi's sarcoma is being seen in greatly increased numbers in patients with acquired immune deficiency syndrome (AIDS). This is more prominent in homosexual males, but much further research is needed to clarify this newly discovered disorder.

HISTOPATHOLOGY FOR THE SURGEON

The surgeon should be aware of the fact that histologic diagnosis may be difficult at times. Characteristic slits (not true blood vessels) within a fibrocytic stroma containing extravasated erythrocytes are one good clue to the diagnosis. In Kaposi's sarcoma with predominant fibrocytic activity, the histopathology has to be differentiated from that of a vascular fibrosarcoma. Surgical treatment and prognosis of the two entities differ greatly.

SURGICAL TREATMENT

It should be mentioned that these tumors are radiosensitive and radiation therapy has been an acceptable treatment for years; however, careful judgment as to when to use this modality should be exercised, since the patient is likely to develop more lesions. If only a few surgically manageable nodules in strategic areas present a problem, surgical excision is an acceptable temporizing method. Only a minimal border is needed when excising these lesions. Circular punches can be quite helpful in this situation. However, surgical treatment or radiation should not be considered curative therapy. Some success has also been achieved with local infiltration and systemic administration of vinca alkaloids.[10]

Since Kaposi's sarcoma associated with AIDS syndrome may behave differently than those cases seen in the past, the methods above may not apply. Further research will help define appropriate treatment for such cases.

REFERENCES

1. Griffith, B. H., and McKinney, P.: An appraisal of treatment of basal cell carcinoma of the skin. Plast Reconstr Surg 51:565, 1973.
2. Pascal, R. R.: Prognosis of "incompletely excised" vs. "completely excised" basal cell carcinoma. Plast Reconstr Surg 41:328, 1968.
3. Lauritzen, R. E., Johnson, R. E., and Spratt, J. S., Jr.: Pattern of recurrence in basal cell carcinoma. Surgery 57:813, 1965.
4. Schultz, B. C., and Roenick, N. H., Jr.: The double scalpel and double punch excision of skin tumors. J Am Acad Dermatol 7:495–599, 1982.
5. Mohs, F. E.: Chemosurgery. Microscopically Controlled Surgery for Skin Cancer. Springfield, Charles C Thomas, 1978.
6. Lund, H. Z.: How often does squamous cell carcinoma of the skin metastasize? Arch Dermatol 92:635, 1965.
7. McPeak, C. J., Cruz, T., and Nicastri, A. D.: Dermatofibrosarcoma protuberans: An analysis of 86 cases—five with metastasis. Ann Surg 166(Suppl 12):803, 1967.
8. Mohs, F. E.: op. cit. p. 219.
9. Bluefarb, S. M.: Kaposis Sarcoma. Springfield, Charles C Thomas, 1959.
10. Tucker, S. B., and Winkelmann, R. K.: Treatment of kaposis sarcoma with vinblastine. Arch Dermatol 112:958, 1976.

Appendix

This section illustrates some common surgical equipment and instruments useful in surgery of the skin. Most are instruments that the authors have used and find helpful in office surgery. Brief comments accompany the illustrations. These illustrations are examples only and are by no means a complete catalogue; nor is the inclusion here of any instrument or device intended to be a recommendation or endorsement of that product. Thorough "hands-on" evaluation of all instruments and equipment is suggested before any purchase is made.

ULTRASONIC CLEANERS

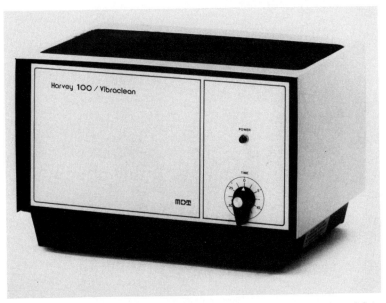

FIGURE A–1. Harvey 100 Vibraclean. It features a simple drain tap and soundproofing lid. It is 14 inches wide by 9 inches high by 10 inches deep. Ultrasonic cleaners are extremely useful in cleaning instruments, especially hard-to-reach places in curves and joints. Instruments should be cleansed of most surface debris before being placed in the ultrasonic cleaner.

SURGICAL LIGHTING

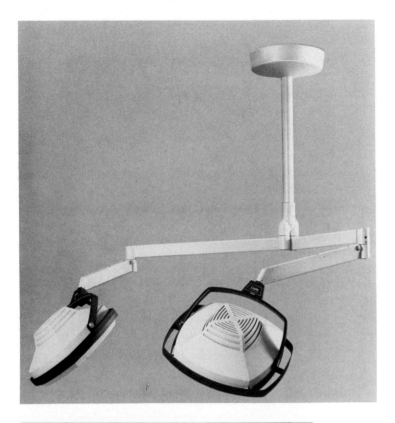

FIGURE A–2. Castle 2420 C minor surgical lights. Each lamp head has an on/off switch. The light is color-corrected and heat-filtered. Each arm rotates 290 degrees, and the center yoke rotates 285 degrees. Each lamp head rotates 180 degrees about its own axis. Sterilizable handles are available.

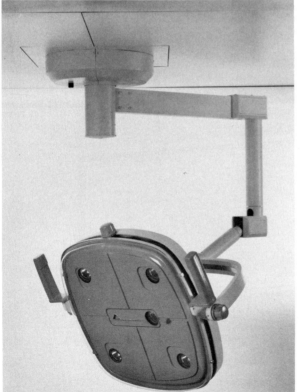

FIGURE A–3. Burton 17102 minor surgical light. Variable adjustments can be made on five 50-watt halogen bulbs. Sterilizable positioning handles and adjustment knobs are included.

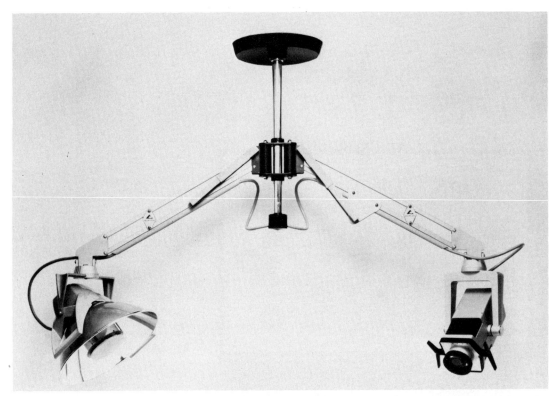

FIGURE A–4. Burton reflector (left) and spotlight (right). Both ceiling and floor mount styles are available. The reflector light is more appropriate and produces less glare for surgical use.

STERILIZERS

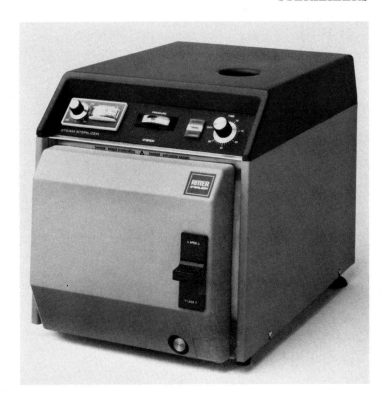

FIGURE A–5. Ritter 800-volt table-top sterilizer. The chamber size is 8 inches by 14½ inches. The average cycle time with two pounds of hard goods is 10 to 14 minutes.

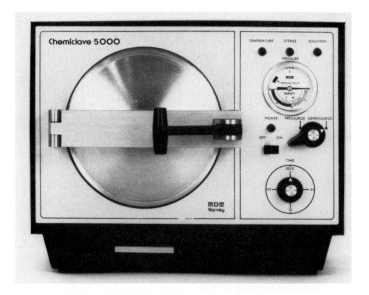

FIGURE A–6. MDT Chemiclave 5000. This uses unsaturated chemical vapor instead of saturated steam. There is less rust, corrosion, and dulling of edges with this method. It has a 20-minute cycle. The chamber size is 6 inches by 11 inches. Some heat-sensitive items (linen, cloth, liquids) cannot be sterilized without damage at the higher temperature (270°F) produced with this form of sterilization.

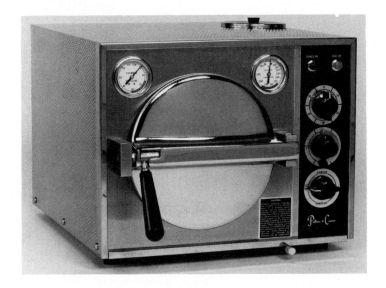

FIGURE A–7. Pelton Crane OCM autoclave. Different chamber sizes are available.

ELECTROSURGERY UNITS

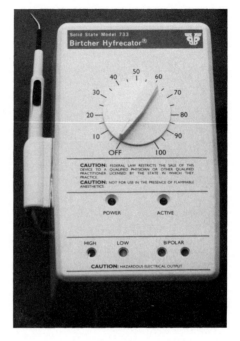

FIGURE A–8. Hyfrecator. This device is used for electrocautery and coagulation. It has no cutting current. It has monopolar and bipolar modes with optional ground plate. A wall bracket is included and a mobile stand is optional. On model 733, a foot control is standard, but an optional handle control is available.

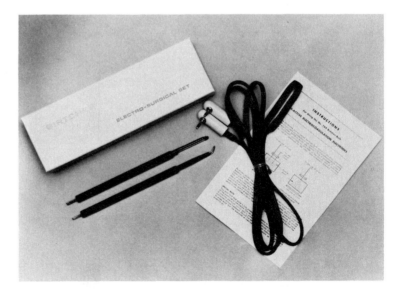

FIGURE A–9. Bi-active electro-coagulation set for use with the Hyfrecator. The current is limited to the area between electrode points and slightly beyond. Current does not travel through the patient to the ground.

TECHNIQUE CONFIGURATIONS

MONOTERMINAL*

For monoterminal fulguration and desiccation procedures, use either the High or Low terminal outputs only. Grounding is achieved by the third wire in the line cord.

The 740, 741 and 744 Sets can be used in this configuration.

MONOPOLAR

This technique delivers power for coagulation from one terminal of an ungrounded bipolar output to a return through the indifferent plate.

The 711A, 711E and 779-3 handles, the 740, 741 and 744 Sets, or forceps may be used in this configuration.

BIPOLAR

Bipolar electrodes actually determine the path of therapeutic current in the area to be coagulated. Bipolar coagulation does not allow current to flow through surrounding organs or tissue.

The 782 and 789 Sets may also be used in this configuration in place of the forceps as shown.

*For international electrical requirements only, a ground jack is provided for use with the dispersive plate in the monoterminal mode.

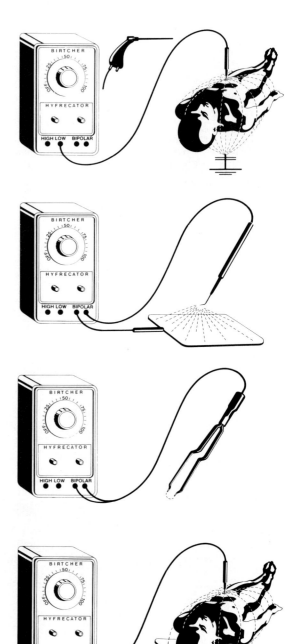

FIGURE A–10. Technique configurations for use with the Hyfrecator.

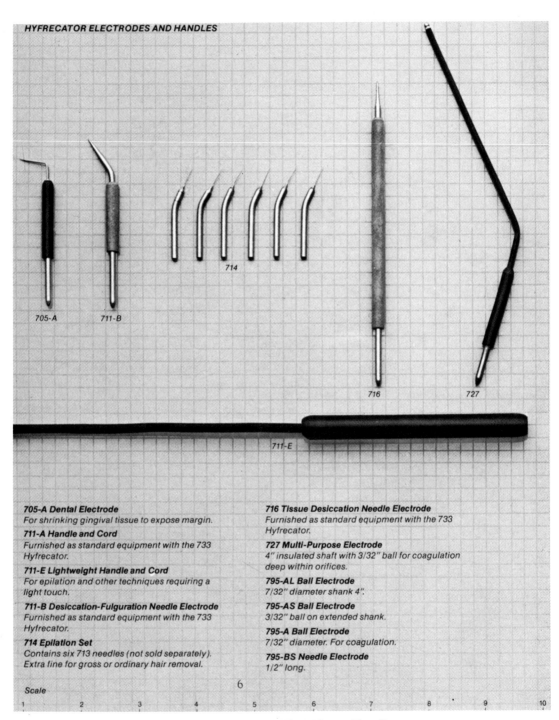

HYFRECATOR ELECTRODES AND HANDLES

705-A   711-B   714   716   727   711-E

705-A Dental Electrode
For shrinking gingival tissue to expose margin.

711-A Handle and Cord
Furnished as standard equipment with the 733 Hyfrecator.

711-E Lightweight Handle and Cord
For epilation and other techniques requiring a light touch.

711-B Desiccation-Fulguration Needle Electrode
Furnished as standard equipment with the 733 Hyfrecator.

714 Epilation Set
Contains six 713 needles (not sold separately). Extra fine for gross or ordinary hair removal.

716 Tissue Desiccation Needle Electrode
Furnished as standard equipment with the 733 Hyfrecator.

727 Multi-Purpose Electrode
4" insulated shaft with 3/32" ball for coagulation deep within orifices.

795-AL Ball Electrode
7/32" diameter shank 4".

795-AS Ball Electrode
3/32" ball on extended shank.

795-A Ball Electrode
7/32" diameter. For coagulation.

795-BS Needle Electrode
1/2" long.

Scale

FIGURE A–11. Hyfrecator electrodes and handles.

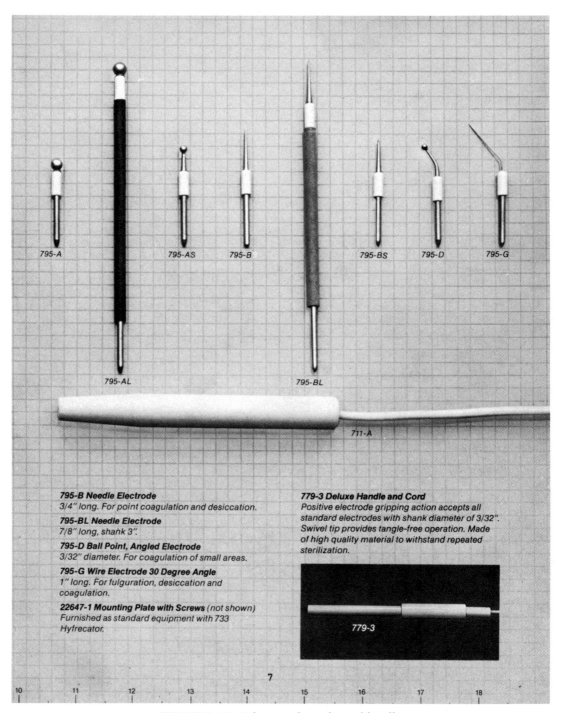

795-A   795-AS   795-B   795-BS   795-D   795-G

795-AL   795-BL

711-A

795-B Needle Electrode
3/4" long. For point coagulation and desiccation.

795-BL Needle Electrode
7/8" long, shank 3".

795-D Ball Point, Angled Electrode
3/32" diameter. For coagulation of small areas.

795-G Wire Electrode 30 Degree Angle
1" long. For fulguration, desiccation and coagulation.

22647-1 Mounting Plate with Screws (not shown)
Furnished as standard equipment with 733 Hyfrecator.

779-3 Deluxe Handle and Cord
Positive electrode gripping action accepts all standard electrodes with shank diameter of 3/32". Swivel tip provides tangle-free operation. Made of high quality material to withstand repeated sterilization.

779-3

7

FIGURE A–12. Hyfrecator electrodes and handles.

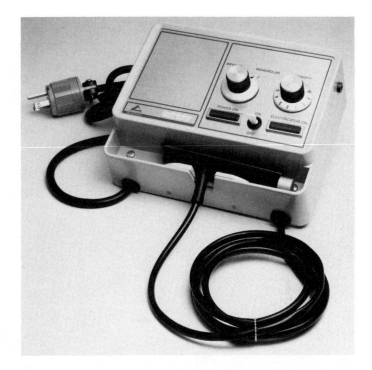

FIGURE A–13. Burton Electricator with hand control. Wall mount and floor stand styles are available. It has both monopolar and bipolar modes. It has no cutting current.

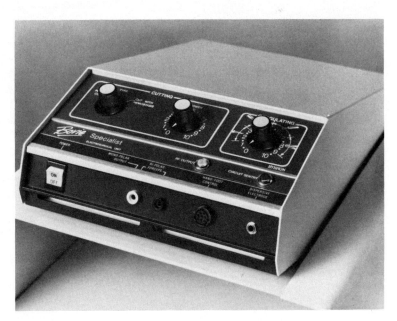

FIGURE A–14. Bovie Specialist electrosurgical unit. It has both cutting and coagulating currents, monopolar and bipolar modes, and hand or foot control.

TABLES

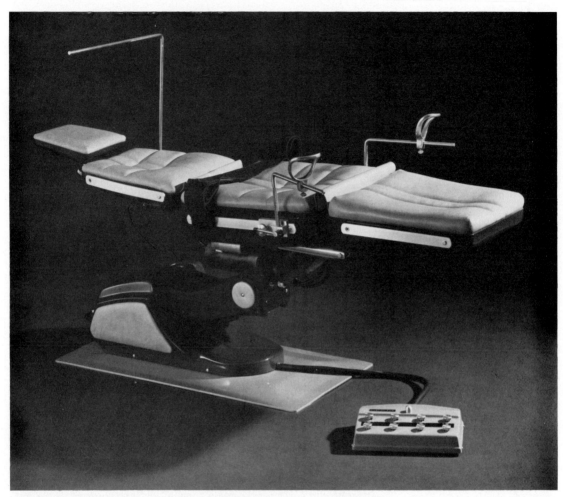

FIGURE A–15. Dexta 50s surgery chair. The seat width is 21½ inches. Accessories include I.V. pole, I.V. arm board, arm-hand surgery board, stirrups, and different power bases for maximum seat heights of 38 to 44½ inches. A paper roll holder may be attached at extra cost.

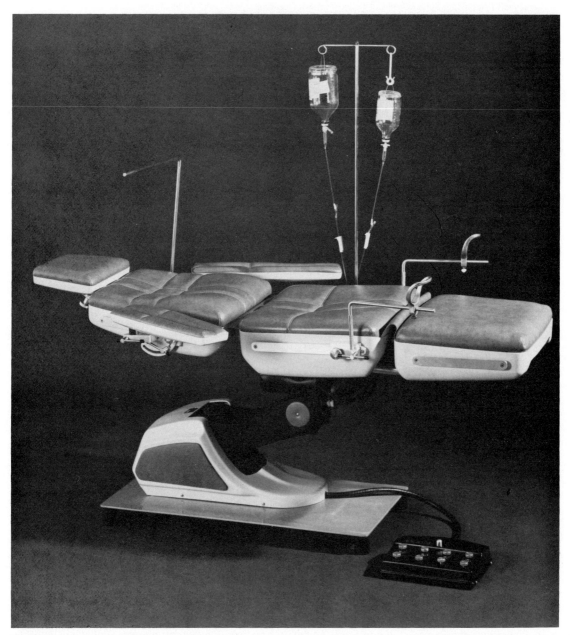

FIGURE A–16. Dexta 52s surgery chair. It is similar to the 50s but 2 inches longer (72 inches) and 2 inches wider (23½ inches). It should be noted that the extra 2-inch width can place substantial additional stress on the surgeon's back when he is operating.

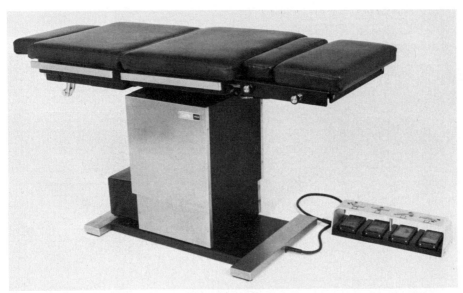

FIGURE A–17. Ritter clinical procedure table. It is wider than previous surgical table series by Ritter. It has an extremely versatile headrest. Plug-in stirrups, paper roll tray and straps, and small drain pan are standard. Options include mobile base and arm board. The table accommodates the proctologic position easily.

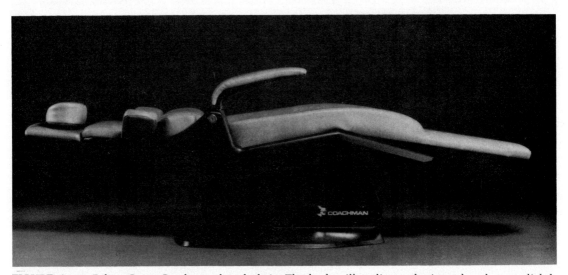

FIGURE A–18. Pelton Crane Coachman dental chair. The back will recline to horizontal and even slightly beyond, almost to the Trendelenburg position. As the back reclines, the foot rest elevates so that an almost flat horizontal position is attainable. There is a foot control and a multifunction switch on the chair back. An articulating headrest is optional. The armrests swing out. The chair is not suitable for gynecologic or proctologic positions. The metal under the armrest should be upholstered to prevent conduction from the electrosurgical unit.

SURGICAL INSTRUMENTS

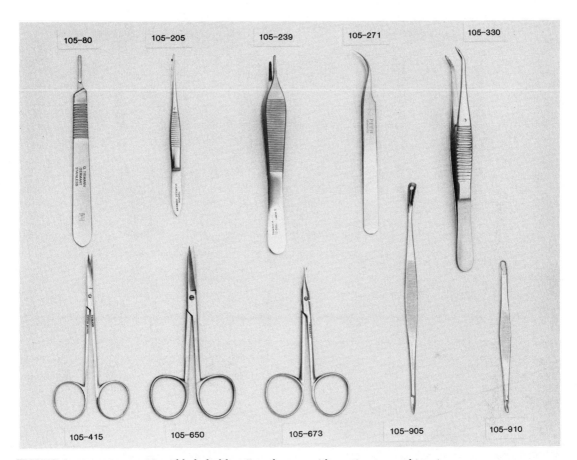

FIGURE A–19. 105–80.   No. 3 blade holder. (I prefer one with centimeter markings.)
105–205. Small tissue forceps with teeth.
105–239. Adson-type tissue forceps.
105–271. Splinter forceps.
105–330. Suture removal forceps. (Note: These pick up fine monofilament sutures very well for easy suture removal.)
105–415. Sharp curved fine iris scissors.
105–650. Straight scissors suitable for suture cutting during surgery.
105–673. Gradle scissors with fine sharp points especially suitable for cutting small lesions (e.g., skin tags).
105–905 and 105–910. Two examples of comedo extractors.

(Courtesy of George Tieman and Company.)

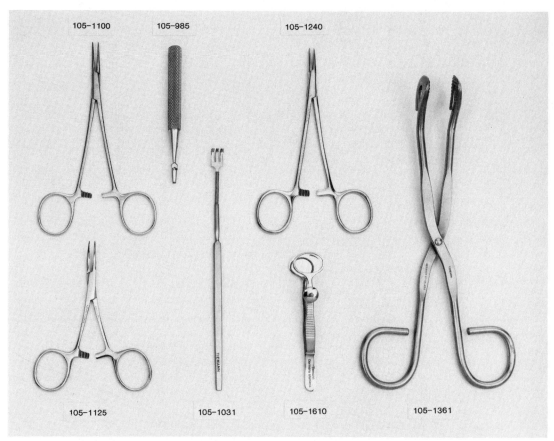

FIGURE A–20. 105–1100. Straight hemostat.
105–985. Keyes-type skin biopsy dermal punch.
105–1240. Short, smooth-jaw Webster-type needle holder suitable for fine, precision-point needles.
105–1125. Curved, small mosquito-type hemostat with fine tips for small blood vessels.
105–1031. Small three-prong, rake-type skin retractor.
105–1610. Small chalazion clamp helpful for immobilizing and promoting pressure hemostasis on eyelids, lips, ala nasi, ear lobes, etc.
105–1361. Sterilizable instrument transfer forceps.

(Courtesy of George Tieman and Company.)

FIGURE A–21. Ethicon precision-point needles. Both needles
have a flat top and bottom beyond the cutting edge to facilitate grasping with a smooth-jaw
needle holder. *Top*, "P" type,
with a sharper point than "cutic-
ular" type needles. The reverse
cutting edge extends back one
third the length of the needle.
Bottom, Cosmetic needle, "Pc"
type, with a finer tip (less metal)
and a conventional cutting edge
for smoother tissue penetration.
The cutting edge is only one
fourth the length of the needle.
(Courtesy of Ethicon.)

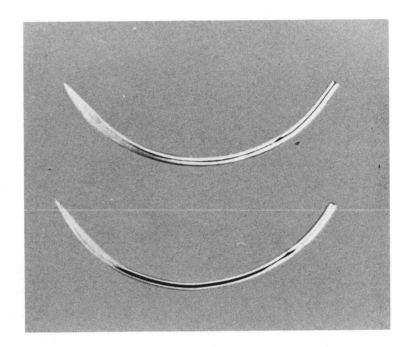

SURGICAL INSTRUMENTS (by Codman)

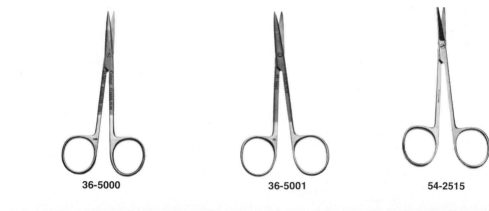

36-5000   **36-5001**   **54-2515**

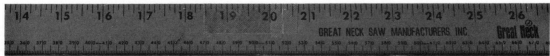

FIGURE A–22. 36–5000. Classic Plus 4-inch straight scissors. (Note: "Classic Plus" instruments are Codman's
top of the line, with a three-year guarantee to "stay like new under normal use."
Codman resharpens and adjusts instruments and replaces inserts if needed under this
guarantee.)
36–5001. Classic Plus 4-inch curved iris scissors.
54–2515. Straight delicate scissors.

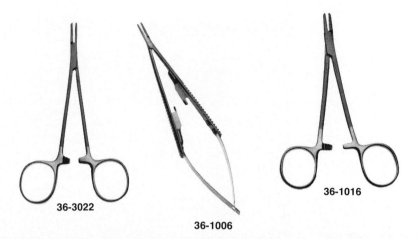

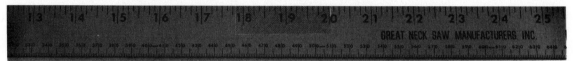

FIGURE A–23. 36–3022. Classic Plus Ryder smooth-jaw needle holder. The jaws are thinner than those of a Halsey or Webster type. This allows more of a needle to be exposed for passage through tissue. This difference may be helpful when using small, precision-type needles. The thinner jaws mean less needle being grasped by the holder and therefore more tendency for the needle to wobble if resistance is met or force exerted. This is an instrument for delicate work.

36–1006. Classic Plus Castroviejo microsurgical smooth-jaw 5-inch needle holder for very delicate work. It is less appropriate for use on skin.

36–1016. Classic Plus Halsey smooth-jaw 5-inch needle holder. This and the Webster smooth jaw are perhaps the most common types used in skin surgery.

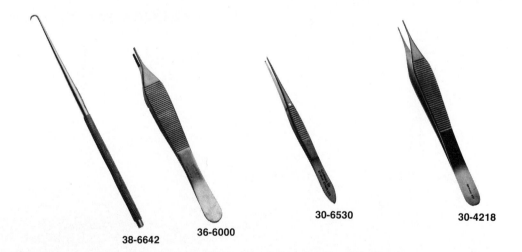

FIGURE A–24. 38–6642. Joseph single-prong skin hook.

36–6000. Classic Plus Adson tissue forceps. Fine serrations on the tungsten carbide jaws enable this device to firmly grab tissue without "teeth." This enables the operator to use dual-purpose tooth and smooth-jaw functions.

30–6530. Straight iris tissue forceps.

30–4218. Delicate Adson tissue forceps.

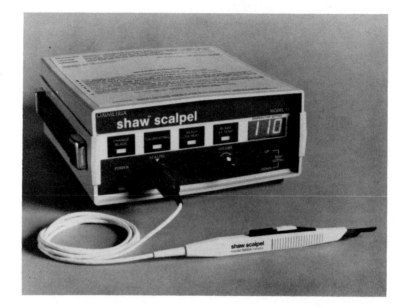

FIGURE A–25. Shaw hot scalpel. Variable adjustment from 110°C to 270°C allows for easy coagulation of blood vessels while cutting.

Index

Page numbers in *italics* refer to figures; page numbers followed by t refer to tables.